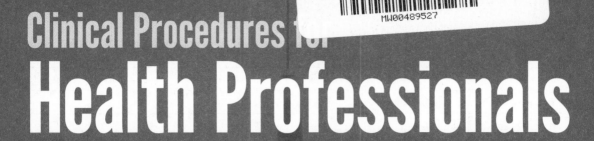

Clinical Procedures for
Health Professionals

Nina Multak, MPAS, PA-C

Associate Clinical Professor, Physician Assistant Department

College of Nursing and Health Professions

Drexel University

Philadelphia, Pennsylvania

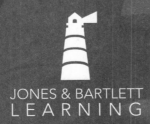

JONES & BARTLETT
LEARNING

World Headquarters
Jones & Bartlett Learning
5 Wall Street
Burlington, MA 01803
978-443-5000
info@jblearning.com
www.jblearning.com

Jones & Bartlett Learning books and products are available through most bookstores and online booksellers. To contact Jones & Bartlett Learning directly, call 800-832-0034, fax 978-443-8000, or visit our website, www.jblearning.com.

Substantial discounts on bulk quantities of Jones & Bartlett Learning publications are available to corporations, professional associations, and other qualified organizations. For details and specific discount information, contact the special sales department at Jones & Bartlett Learning via the above contact information or send an email to specialsales@jblearning.com.

7862-3

Production Credits

VP, Executive Publisher: David D. Cella
Executive Acquisitions Editor: Nancy Anastasi Duffy
Editorial Assistant: Jade Freeman
Associate Director of Production: Julie C. Bolduc
Production Manager: Daniel Stone
Associate Production Editor: Brooke Appe
Marketing Manager: Grace Richards
Manufacturing and Inventory Control Supervisor: Amy Bacus
Composition: S4Carlisle Publishing Services

Cover Design: Michael O'Donnell
Associate Director of Rights & Media: Joanna Lundeen
Rights & Media Specialist: Wes DeShano
Rights & Media Database Coordinator: Mike Wile
Media Development Editor: Shannon Sheehan
Media Development Editor: Troy Liston
Cover Image: © nito/Shutterstock
Printing and Binding: Edwards Brothers Malloy
Cover Printing: Edwards Brothers Malloy

Library of Congress Cataloging-in-Publication Data
Clinical procedures for health professionals / edited by Nina Multak.
    p. ; cm.
Includes bibliographical references.
ISBN 978-1-284-03241-3 (pbk. : alk. paper)
I. Multak, Nina, editor.
[DNLM: 1. Therapeutics--methods. 2. Clinical Competence. 3. Diagnostic Techniques and Procedures. WB 300]
RC71.3
616.07'5--dc23
                    2015035241

6048

Printed in the United States of America
19 18 17 16   10 9 8 7 6 5 4 3 2

Acknowledgements

I would like to express my gratitude to my family, colleagues, friends, and students.

To my family: Alex, Ariel, Ilana and Ben, Thank for your inspiration, enthusiastic encouragement, and love. To my siblings Alisa, David, and your families, thank you for your never-ending support. Lastly, thank you to my parents, Beverly and Simeon, for a lifetime of continuous encouragement.

To my colleagues and friends: Your teamwork, skill, and dedication are unparalleled! I am grateful to work with such a fine group of individuals. To Patrick C. Auth, my sincere gratitude for your support and constructive suggestions during the planning and development of this project.

I would also like to thank Jade Freeman, Brooke Appe, Wesley DeShano, and Teresa Reilly from Jones & Bartlett Learning for your valuable advice and wonderful assistance throughout this project.

To my students: Your dedication to providing high caliber patient care was the inspiration for this resource.

Nina L. Multak

Brief Contents

Brief Contents continued

Contents

Contents continued

Contents continued

Contents continued

Contents continued

Preface

In compiling this resource we wanted to provide students with rapid access to information they need in the clinical environment. Using current technology, students can immediately access information describing and demonstrating clinical procedures. This resource can be used in both inpatient and ambulatory environments to help student clinicians perform procedures accurately and safely. We envision students viewing clinical procedures on their mobile devices to review the information learned in the classroom setting prior to performing a procedure on their next patient. While we acknowledge that this resource does not contain a description of every procedure required of a student clinician, it contains a very comprehensive selection of procedures.

To provide instant access to this information, we turned to experienced clinician educators from various healthcare professions. Contributors to this resource include nurses, advanced practice nurses, nurse anesthetists, physician assistants, and physicians. All of the videos include mannequin simulators or task trainers for demonstration. It is recommended that students practice these procedures under the guidance of an instructor or practicing clinician prior to performing these procedures on their patients.

We hope that by using this resource, each student is supported by information at their fingertips which gives them the confidence and skill needed to perform each procedure safely.

About the Editor

Nina Multak, MPAS, PA-C is an Associate Clinical Professor in the Physician Assistant Department, College of Nursing and Health Professions at Drexel University. She is a Distinguished Fellow of the American Academy of Physician Assistants and a certified physician assistant. Nina Multak is a doctoral candidate in the Drexel University College of Computing and Informatics. Current research includes health information technology, healthcare simulation, and inter-professional education. She has held previous faculty appointments at the University of Florida College of Medicine, NOVA Southeastern University, and the Philadelphia College of Osteopathic Medicine. She is a graduate of the Hahnemann University Physician Assistant Program. Her Masters in Physician Assistant Studies was awarded from the University of Nebraska with an emphasis on educational innovation for physician assistant students.

Nina Multak maintains professional affiliations with the American Academy of Physician Assistants, Pennsylvania Academy of Physician Assistants, Physician Assistant Education Association, Society for Simulation in Healthcare, and the American Society for Information Science and Technology. She has lectured at the local, state, national, and international levels. Additionally, she has authored textbook chapters and has published journal articles on topics in healthcare, utilization of mannequin simulators and standardized patients in physician assistant training programs, and health information exchange.

Contributors

Patrick Auth, PhD, MS, PA-C
Clinical Professor
Chair, Physician Assistant Department
Drexel University
College of Nursing and Health Professions
Philadelphia, Pennsylvania

Adrian Banning, MMS, PA-C
Assistant Clinical Professor
Drexel University
College of Nursing and Health Professions
Philadelphia, Pennsylvania

Lew Bennett, CRNA, DNP
Assistant Clinical Professor
Chair, Nurse Anesthesia Program
Drexel University
College of Nursing and Health Professions
Philadelphia, Pennsylvania

Jim Burkett, MS, EMT-P, PA-C
Assistant Professor
Director, Advanced Physician Assistant Degree
Program
A.T. Still University
Mesa, Arizona

Nikhil Chawla, MD
Drexel University
College of Medicine
Philadelphia, Pennsylvania

Ferne Cohen, MSN, CRNA, EdD
Assistant Clinical Professor
Associate Director, Nurse Anesthesia Program
Drexel University
College of Nursing and Health Professions
Philadelphia, Pennsylvania

James Connolly, MD
Drexel University
College of Medicine
Philadelphia, Pennsylvania

John Cornele, MSN, RN, CNE, EMT-P
Director, Center for Interdisciplinary Clinical
Simulation and Practice
Drexel University
College of Nursing and Health Professions
Philadelphia, Pennsylvania

Rosalie Coppola, MHS, PA-C
Associate Clinical Professor
Drexel University
College of Nursing and Health Professions
Philadelphia, Pennsylvania

Joseph DiChiara, DO
Drexel University
College of Medicine
Philadelphia, Pennsylvania

Contributors continued

Michael Green, DO
Chair and Program Director, Anesthesia
Department
Associate Professor
Hahnemann University Hospital
Drexel University
College of Medicine
Philadelphia, Pennsylvania

Sharon Griswold-Theodorson, MD, MPH
Director, Simulation Division, Department
  of EM
Director, Master's Degree in Medical/Healthcare
  Simulation
Professor
Drexel University
College of Medicine
Philadelphia, Pennsylvania

Michelle Heinan, EdD, PA-C
Director, Physician Assistant Program
Concordia University
Mequon, Wisconsin

Nancy Hurwitz, PA-C, MHP
Assistant Professor
School of Physician Assistant Studies
Boston, Massachusetts

Abby Jacobson, MS, PA-C
Family Dermatology of Reading
Reading, Pennsylvania
Assistant Professor
Salus University
Elkins Park, Pennsylvania

Lisa A. Johnson, DrNP, CRNP, ACNP-BC
Assistant Professor
DeSales University
Department of Nursing and Health
Center Valley, Pennsylvania

Misty Kagarise, DHSc, PA-C, CLS
Associate Professor
Master of Medical Science/Master of Health
Science Programs
Saint Francis University
Loretto, Pennsylvania

Joshua Lenchus, DO, RPh, FACP, SFHM
Associate Professor of Clinical Medicine and
Anesthesiology
University of Miami
Miller School of Medicine
Miami, Florida

Daniela Livingston, MD, PA-C
Assistant Clinical Professor
Drexel University
College of Nursing and Health Professions
Philadelphia, Pennsylvania

Maha B. Lund, DHSc, PA-C
Director, Physician Assistant Program
Department of Family and Preventive Medicine
Emory University School of Medicine
Atlanta, Georgia

Mary Mahabee-Betts, BSN, RN, CNOR
Clinical Nurse Specialist
Temple University Hospital
Philadelphia, Pennsylvania

Kate Morse, PhD, CRNP-BC, CNE, CCRN
Center for Medical Simulation
Harvard University
Boston, Massachusetts

Nina Multak, PhD (c), MPAS, PA-C
Associate Clinical Professor
Drexel University
College of Nursing and Health Professions
Philadelphia, Pennsylvania

Carol Okupniak, DNP, RN-BC
Assistant Clinical Professor of Nursing
Drexel University
College of Nursing and Health Professions
Philadelphia, Pennsylvania

**Deborah A. Opacic, MMS, EdD, PA-C,
DFAAPA**
Assistant Professor
Director, Physician Assistant Studies
University of Pittsburgh
Pittsburgh, Pennsylvania

Jessica Parsons, MD
Assistant Professor
Associate Director, Emergency Medicine
Residency Program
Drexel University
College of Medicine
Philadelphia, Pennsylvania

Jill Sanko, PhD, MS, ARNP, CHSE-A
Assistant Professor
Academic and Research Director of Simulation
University of Miami School of Nursing and
   Health Studies
Miami, Florida

Poovendran Saththasivam, MD
Drexel University
College of Medicine
Philadelphia, Pennsylvania

Jami S. Smith, MEd, MPA, PA-C
Academic Director
Master of Science in Medical and Healthcare
Simulation Program
Department of Emergency Medicine
Drexel University
College of Medicine
Philadelphia, Pennsylvania

Charles Stream, MHS, PA-C
Anesthesia Associates of Lancaster
Lancaster, Pennsylvania

**Linda Wilson, RN, PhD, CPAN, CAPA, BC,
CNE, CHSE, CHSE-A, ANEF, FAAN**
Clinical Professor
Assistant Dean for Special Projects, Simulation
and CNE Accreditation & Associate
Drexel University
College of Nursing and Health Professions
Philadelphia, Pennsylvania

UNIT 1

CORE PROCEDURES

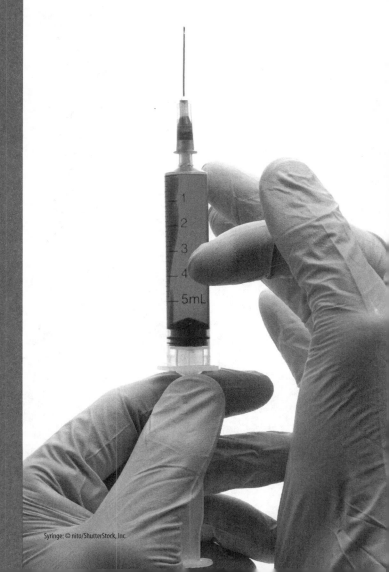

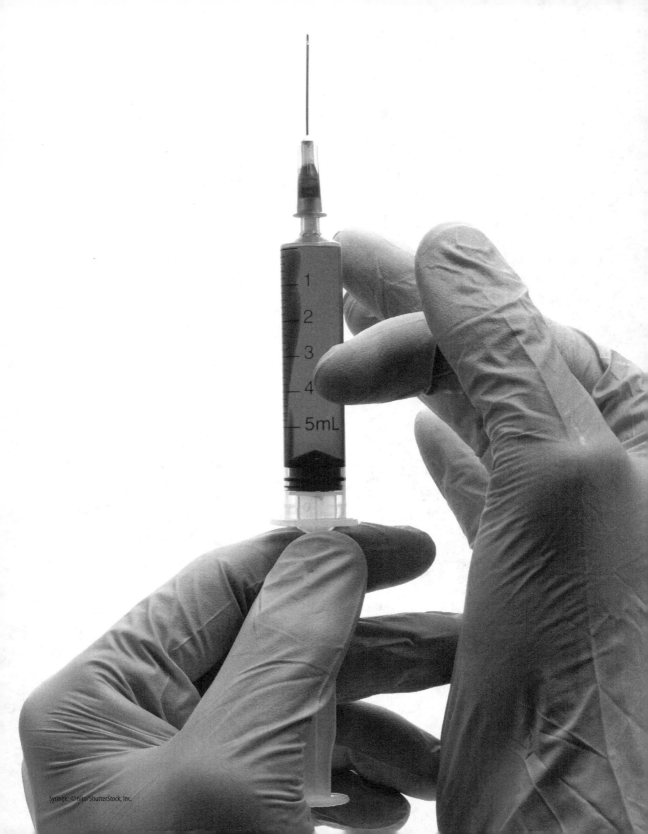

CHAPTER 1

Aseptic Technique

Jill Sanko, PhD, MS, ARNP, CHSE-A
Joshua D. Lenchus, DO, RPh, FACP, SFHM

GOALS

▶ Identify the steps necessary to achieve and preserve a sterile field for invasive procedures taking place outside of an operating room or interventional suite.

▶ Highlight the knowledge and performance steps needed to achieve asepsis.

▶ Gain the knowledge necessary for aseptic technique and understand information on the performance elements necessary for achieving asepsis when performing invasive procedures.

▶ Achieve and maintain a sterile field.

▶ Properly break down a field.

▶ Remove **personal protective equipment** following completion of a procedure.

OBJECTIVES

1. Recognize the importance of asepsis during invasive procedures and its role in patient safety.
2. Appreciate the value and importance of proper hand hygiene before and after the performance of an invasive procedure.
3. Examine the importance of creating and maintaining a sterile field.
4. Determine the utility, relevance, and applicability of full sterile protective clothing.
5. Contrast "clean technique" with "aseptic technique."
6. Employ sterile technique while putting on appropriate personal protective equipment (e.g., face mask, cap, gown, gloves).
7. Perform the correct method for preparing and draping a sterile field for commonly performed bedside procedures.
8. Manage a break in aseptic technique.
9. Demonstrate the removal of personal protective equipment.
10. Illustrate how to safely dispose of sharps post-procedure.

RATIONALE

- **Asepsis** is the state of being free from living pathogenic microorganisms (e.g., bacteria, viruses, fungi, and parasites) that have the possibility of causing disease or illness.
- There are two categories of asepsis: (1) general asepsis, which applies to patient care procedures outside an operating room, and (2) surgical asepsis, which is related to those procedures that take place within an operating room and is designed to prevent surgical site infections. The scope of this chapter focuses on the establishment of general asepsis.[i]
- Establishing and maintaining asepsis is a vital first step for all invasive procedures. Failure to protect patients undergoing invasive procedures through the creation of a germ-free, safe area in which to complete a procedure may lead to life-threatening illnesses or death. Fortunately, general asepsis and environmentally safe areas can be easily attained and maintained by learning the steps outlined in this chapter.

EVIDENCE-BASED INDICATIONS

- Infections acquired during a hospital stay, regardless of the mechanism of cause, are known as **healthcare-associated** infections (HAIs). Strict adherence to proper hand hygiene among healthcare providers and proper assignment of clean, sterile, and aseptic techniques appropriate for procedures performed on patients are important in the prevention of HAIs. These infections significantly affect patient safety, costs associated with hospital care, and morbidity and mortality of patients.
- It has been estimated that upwards of 1.7 million HAIs are acquired annually by patients hospitalized in the United States, and HAI is among the leading causes of preventable deaths in the United States.[1] According to the U.S. Department of Health and Human Services (HHS), HAIs alone are responsible for $28–33 billion in preventable healthcare expenditures each year.[2]

Numerous types of aseptic techniques are utilized in bedside and surgical suite settings. **TABLE 1-1** provides information for the most commonly used aseptic techniques. In general the approach taken is dictated by the planned procedure.

- Aseptic technique is a stepwise approach to the construction and continuation of a sterile field (an area free of disease-causing microorganisms) in which the performance of any procedure that will create or expose a break in the skin's integrity can be safely performed. Included in this chapter are information and supplemental tools that will assist in the instruction and understanding of aseptic technique for bedside procedures.
- These tools include:
  - A mnemonic that can facilitate recall in planning for the preparation of oneself and the sterile field
  - A checklist that can also be used for recall and planning or for evaluating performance
  - Numerous charts

CONTRAINDICATIONS

None

COMPLICATIONS

- Unavailable supplies may lead to infection. For example, if **chlorhexidine** is not available and alcohol is used as a substitute during a central line placement, the patient may contract an infection.
- Break in sterile technique (see **TABLE 1-2**).

PLANNING FOR THE PROCEDURE

- Proper planning is an important first step in establishing any procedural environment; the acronym SCRIPT[4] can aid in remembering initial considerations for a variety of procedural conditions (see **BOX 1-1**).

TABLE 1-1: Types of Techniques

	Clean Technique	Modified Aseptic Technique	Aseptic Technique	Surgical Asepsis
Goal	Reduction of transient* microorganisms	Reduction of transient microorganisms	Elimination of transient microorganisms	Elimination of transient and resident[†] microorganisms
Setting	Any healthcare area	Bedside or procedure area	Bedside or procedure area	Operating room
Examples of Procedures	Taking blood pressure or temperature, feeding a patient, general examination	Peripheral intravenous line placement, routine phlebotomy, intubation	Central venous catheter placement, paracentesis, lumbar puncture	Surgical procedure
Hand Hygiene	Routine[‡]	Routine[‡]	Routine[‡]	Surgical scrub
Personal Protective Equipment	None usually	Mask and face shield or goggles if splashing is a possibility	Hat, mask with/without face shield, sterile gown	Hat, mask with/without face shield, sterile gown
Glove Type	None or clean	Clean	Sterile	Sterile
Field	None	Clean area	Sterile field	Sterile field
Patient/Site Prep	None	None or alcohol	Chlorhexidine or Povidone-iodine	Chlorhexidine or Povidone-iodine

*Transient microorganisms are those that are found in the environment and are picked up on the hands of healthcare workers (HCWs) during the course of routine daily work. These types of organisms do not generally take up permanent residence as normal flora.
[†]Resident microorganisms are those that are found as normal flora on the hands of HCWs.
[‡]In healthcare settings, hand hygiene should be performed with an antimicrobial soap.

TABLE 1-2: Types of Breaks in Peri-procedural Sterile Technique

Breaks in sterile technique can be divided into the following four types:[3]

- Type 1—Immediate recognition
- Type 2—Recognition shortly after it occurs
- Type 3—Delayed recognition
- Type 4—Unrecognized (noted after completion of the procedure)

BOX 1-1: SCRIPT

Space and workflow?
Clean, aseptic, or sterile technique?
Routine, aseptic, or surgical hand hygiene?
Instruments and supplies?
Personal protective equipment?
Trash: sharps, infectious waste, radioactive waste, pathology waste, or routine waste?

- A checklist is another tool that can aid in remembering crucial steps in a complex procedure. Research supports the use of checklists when completing multiple-step tasks such as the establishment of a procedural environment. According to Hales and Pronovost, the checklist is an important tool in error management and contributes significantly to reducing the risk of costly mistakes and the improvement of overall outcomes.[3] A checklist, such as the one developed by the procedure program at the University of Miami-Jackson Memorial Hospital Center for Patient Safety,[5] may also serve as a valuable tool for learning the proper steps in preparing for invasive bedside procedures, and for ensuring that no steps are missed.

PROCEDURAL INSTRUCTIONS

- This section addresses each of the steps as listed in the gowning, gloving, and aseptic technique checklist presented in the supplemental materials for this chapter; steps are listed in chronological order.

Step 1: Obtain the Proper Personal Protective Equipment (PPE) for the Planned Procedure

- Full PPE is necessary for many of the invasive procedures that are performed outside a surgical suite and includes hat, mask (with or without a face shield), goggles (if no face shield), a sterile gown, gloves (sterile or clean), and draping materials.

- All materials should be obtained and present at the bedside prior to beginning the procedure. Leaving the environment to obtain missing items may lead to a break in asepsis.
- Proper training and education in the correct use of PPE are required per **Occupational Safety and Health Administration (OSHA)** standards.[5] Such training should include the following:
  - When PPE is necessary
  - What PPE is necessary
  - How to properly put on, take off, adjust, and wear the PPE
  - The limitations of PPE
  - Proper care, maintenance, useful life, and disposal of PPE
- Employers should make sure that each employee demonstrates an understanding of the PPE training and the ability to properly wear and use PPE before he or she is allowed to perform work requiring the use of PPE.
- The primary roles of PPE are to protect staff, reduce opportunities for transmission of microorganisms in hospitals, and reduce infection in patients.[6] Prior to beginning any procedure, a hazard assessment is recommended to establish exposure risk for the healthcare provider, as well as the infection transmission risk for the patient, in order to determine the proper PPE needed for the procedure planned. Such a hazard assessment should include a survey of the following:
  - Does the patient's infectious disease status pose a risk to the healthcare provider or other patients?
  - Is the patient immunocompetent or immunocompromised?
  - Is body fluid exposure possible or likely?
  - Is there a risk of a needlestick injury, or will sharp instruments be used?
- There are common and customary PPE for most invasive bedside procedures. **TABLE 1-3** presents required PPE for a variety of procedures that occur at a patient's bedside.

TABLE 1-3: PPE Requirements for Common Procedures

Procedure	Hat	Mask	Face Shield	Sterile Gown	Glove	Draping
Peripheral intravenous line placement, routine phlebotomy	No	No	No	No	Clean	Clean Chux
Arterial line placement	Yes	Yes	Yes	Yes	Sterile	Local area
Central venous catheter insertion	Yes	Yes	Yes	Yes	Sterile	Full maximum barrier
Paracentesis	Yes	Yes	Yes	Yes	Sterile (optional)	Local area
Thoracentesis, pericardiocentesis	Yes	Yes	Yes	Yes	Sterile	Local area
Bone marrow aspiration	No	No	No	No	Sterile	Local area
Joint aspiration	No	No	No	No	Sterile	Local area
Lumbar puncture, ventriculostomy, and intracranial pressure monitor insertion	Yes	Yes	Yes	Yes	Sterile	Local area
Indwelling urinary catheter insertion	No	Recommended	Recommended	No	Sterile	Local area

Step 2: Obtain Proper Antiseptic for the Procedure

- Skin antisepsis is the process of applying a cleaning agent to the patient's skin in order to eliminate transient microorganisms and reduce resident skin flora that may present an infection risk if transferred to the bloodstream. Selecting the appropriate agent will depend on the procedure, patient sensitivities or allergies, and its institutional availability.

- Chlorhexidine[ii] has gained popularity as a **skin antiseptic** since the 1970s. It has several advantages over the more traditional povidone-iodine solutions. Chlorhexidine is applied in repeated back-and-forth strokes, going over the same area multiple times, akin to applying several coats of paint. In contrast, povidone-iodine is applied in outwardly concentric circles, never going over the same area more than once. Chlorhexidine does not pose a risk of skin irritation or allergic reaction like povidone-iodine solutions and, therefore, does not need to be removed following completion of the procedure. Lastly, chlorhexidine appears to have superior skin antisepsis efficacy. A meta-analysis compared the use of chlorhexidine gluconate with povidone-iodine solution in preventing catheter-related bloodstream infections and found the incidence of bloodstream infections was significantly reduced in patients who underwent site preparation with chlorhexidine gluconate versus povidone-iodine.[7] However, chlorhexidine is not appropriate for every procedure, so care must be taken to select the correct agent for the procedure being performed. **TABLE 1-4** presents skin-prep agents used for common procedures.

Step 3: Obtain Proper Kit or Supplies for the Procedure Planned

- Select an appropriate kit or supplies for the procedure planned, paying close attention to size requirements based on the age and size of your patient, as applicable.

Step 4: Prepare a Proper Working Surface

- Having a clean table on which to place needed equipment and the procedural kit facilitates completion of the procedure in a way that is safe for the patient and the healthcare provider. The common practice of using the sterile field may not be the best area to place all the items you will need. Patient movements can sometimes cause items to fall and subsequently become contaminated. A bedside table or instrument stand is commonly used and is a readily available alternative to using the patient or his/her bed as a holding area for equipment. If a bedside table or instrument stand is used, it should be clean, dry, and prepared appropriately for the sterile or clean procedure.

Step 5: Put on Hat

- Surgical hats or caps should be used for those procedures for which full PPE is required (see Table 1-3). Use of a hat or cap prevents the healthcare provider's hair from falling onto the sterile field and contaminating it. Surgical or bouffant type, disposable, or reusable hats are all acceptable choices.

TABLE 1-4: Skin Prep Agents for Common Procedures

Procedure	Skin Prep Agent
Peripheral intravenous line	Alcohol acceptable, but chlorhexidine may have superior infection protection
Indwelling urinary catheter	Povidone-iodine
Routine phlebotomy	Alcohol acceptable, but chlorhexidine may have superior infection protection
Central venous catheter	Chlorhexidine-gluconate
Lumbar puncture	Povidone-iodine
Thoracentesis, paracentesis, and most other invasive procedures	Povidone-iodine acceptable, but chlorhexidine has been shown to have superior infection protection

FIGURE 1-1: Place hat

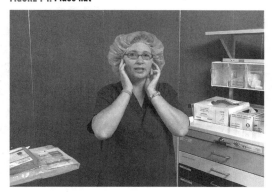

FIGURE 1-2: Place mask

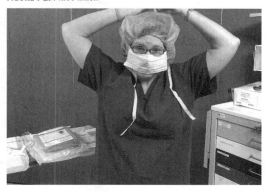

FIGURE 1-3: Tie mask

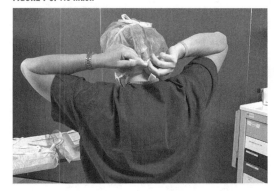

- Donning of a hat or scrub cap is simple (see **FIGURE 1-1**). Place the hat or cap over the head, ensuring that all hair is tucked into the hat; providers with long hair may need to secure their hair prior to donning the hat. If there are ties, they should be comfortably secured at the back.

Step 6: Put on Mask

- Masks should be worn for all procedures for which full PPE is indicated (see Table 1-3). If splashing or spraying of bodily fluids is likely, a face shield or goggles should be worn. Masks prevent microorganisms from transferring to the patient from the healthcare provider's mouth or nasopharynx during talking, coughing, or sneezing. Further, masks and face shields offer protection for the provider in the event of a bodily fluid splash or spray.
- Masks should be secured comfortably by tying both sets of ties, one at the top of the head and one along the nape of the neck or looping earpieces over the ears (see **FIGURES 1-2** and **1-3**). The nosepiece of the mask should be gently pinched at the bridge of the nose to create a tapered area where the mask covers the nose. The bottom aspect of the mask should be pulled down below the chin and any facial hair. If goggles are being used, they should fit snugly over

FIGURE 1-4: Place eye protection

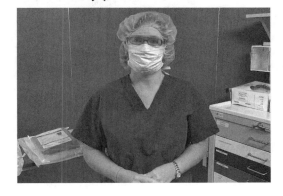

and around the eyes (see **FIGURE 1-4**). Personal eyeglasses are not a sufficient substitute for goggles. If eyeglasses are worn, goggles can be fitted over them.

Step 7: Prepare and Position the Patient for Comfort and for the Procedure Being Performed

- Draping requirements and positioning for various procedures can sometimes be uncomfortable for the patient. Verbally prepare the patient for what to expect and ensure that he or she is as comfortable as possible, while still in the best position for the procedure (see **FIGURE 1-5**).
- For procedures that require the face and head to be draped, one should discuss any potential issues with this preparation (e.g., claustrophobia). Drapes can often be tented to create room between the patient's face and the drape, which can lessen the feeling of enclosure. But, sterility of the site must be maintained.

FIGURE 1-5: Prepare and position patient

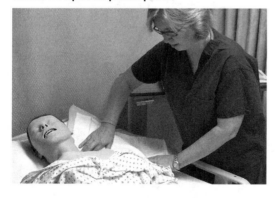

Step 8: Wash Hands

- Handwashing is a critical step in the prevention of HAIs. Prior to beginning any invasive procedure, providers should thoroughly wash their hands with a broad-spectrum antimicrobial agent with the goal being hand antisepsis (see **FIGURE 1-6**).[8,9]
- Ideally, handwashing prior to performing an invasive procedure should include removal

FIGURE 1-6: Wash hands

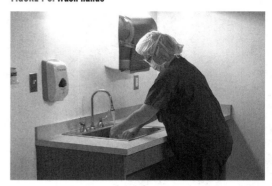

of rings, watches, and bracelets and begin with removal of debris from underneath the fingernails using a nail cleaner. Next, vigorously rub all surfaces of the hands and fingers up to 2–3 inches above the wrists, taking care to angle the hands upward so that dirty water runs down the arms toward the elbows and away from clean surfaces. Scrub time should be at least 15–20 seconds. Hands should be rinsed completely to remove residual soap and then dried with clean single-use paper towels. Faucets should be shut off using a clean paper towel to avoid recontamination of hands. If a sink is not available, an alcohol-based hand rub may be used. A scrub with this type of agent should be done for at least 15–20 seconds.

- Gowning and gloving should take place within 1–2 minutes of completing hand hygiene. Touching of potentially contaminated surfaces should not be done between hand hygiene and donning of PPE. **TABLE 1-5** contains information on required hand hygiene for conditions encountered by healthcare providers caring for patients.

Step 9: Dry Hands

- Following handwashing, hands should be thoroughly dried using a clean single-use paper towel, taking care to dry between fingers (see **FIGURE 1-7**). A patting, rather than

TABLE 1-5: Types of Hand Care

	Purpose	Method
Hand Wash	To remove soil, visible dirt, and transient microorganisms	Soap or detergent for at least 10–15 seconds
Hand Antisepsis	To remove and/or destroy transient microorganisms	Antimicrobial soap or detergent, or alcohol-based hand rub for at least 10–15 seconds
Surgical Hand Scrub	To remove and/or destroy transient microorganisms and reduce resident flora	Antimicrobial soap or detergent preparation with brush to achieve friction for at least 120 seconds, or alcohol-based preparation designed for surgical hand antisepsis*

Source: Larsen EL. APIC guideline for handwashing and hand antisepsis in health care settings. *Am J Infect Control.* 1995 Aug;23(4):251–69.
Purell® surgical scrub requires a two-step application with dry time between each application.

a rubbing, motion should be employed when drying hands to avoid friction on the skin, which can cause breakdown. The paper towel included with most sterile gowns should be used for this purpose if this gown is required PPE.

- If an alcohol-based hand rub is used, care should be taken to allow for the agent to completely dry prior to donning PPE.

Step 10: Don Gown

- Gowning is best done with the help of an assistant. The assistant may open the package and remove the gown in an upward motion, freeing it from its packaging. Next, the gown should be held at the neck band on the inside of the gown. Then, the assistant should step back from the procedure table or area to an unobstructed space and allow the gown to partially unfold (without coming into contact with any unsterile surfaces); if the gown does not completely unfold, a second assistant can pull the bottom of the gown by grasping the inside bottom of

FIGURE 1-7: Dry hands

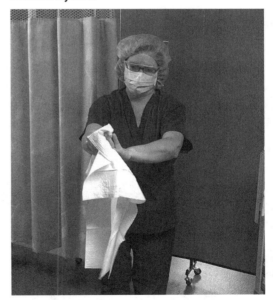

the gown and guiding it down. The inside of the gown should remain in front of the person donning it. Arms should enter first, extended straight out in front, and remain at shoulder height while entering the gown. If the open glove technique is employed, the hands should exit the sleeve cuffs to the point of the wrist. If, however, the closed glove method is being employed, the hands should remain mostly within the cuffs of the sleeves, exiting only to the point of the thumbs (see **FIGURE 1-8**).

FIGURE 1-8: Don gown

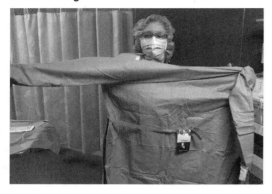

- If an assistant is not being used, remove the gown from the package, grasping the gown on the inside at the armholes, step back to a clear area, free of any obstructions. Next, gently shake the gown to unfold it. Once it is unfolded, enter the gown one arm at a time taking care to keep the arms extended straight out, or up toward the ceiling, being careful not to touch anything (see **FIGURE 1-9**).

FIGURE 1-9: Don gown

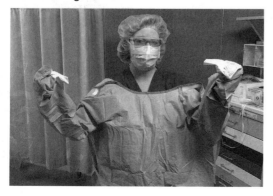

Step 11: Fasten the Gown with the Help of an Assistant

- Once the gown is donned, an assistant pulls the gown up and over the shoulders of the gowned person and fastens the neckband. Next, the inner waist ties are carefully secured, such that the inner aspect of the gown is the only surface handled. Following donning of sterile gloves (see next section), the person wearing the gown grasps the tie card (in the area indicated on the card) at the front of the gown that holds the outer ties, separates the left tie from the card, and holds it in his or her left hand. The card is then handed to the assistant, who grabs the card in the indicated area. Next, the scrubbed person turns to the right, completing the turn when his or her front is facing the assistant. The assistant extends the right tie to its full length, and the gowned person grasps it and ties the left and right ties together at the waist on the left.

Step 12: Don Gloves

- Choose either sterile or clean gloves depending on the procedure being performed. Choosing the appropriate glove size is important. Clean gloves come in extra small, small, medium, and large, while sterile gloves come in numbered sizes from 5.5 to 9, with 5.5 being the smallest. Both clean and sterile gloves come in latex and non-latex varieties. Choose one based on the sensitivities or allergies of the patient and healthcare provider.
- For sterile gloves:
  - Open the outer package of gloves, laying the inner package on a flat surface, and carefully open the right and left sides of the package to expose the gloves. There is a 1-inch "safety margin" at the folded edge of the packaging that can be used to pull open the package. While opening the inner package, take care to touch only the outside edge of the paper and ensure that it stays open by gently bending the flaps out and down as they are opened. The

gloves should be positioned with the cuff openings facing the gowned person.

- To start, choose either the right or left hand (depending on which is the dominant hand) and apply the glove in front of the hand that will be gloved first. If the closed glove method is being used, grasp the cuff of the glove with the nondominant hand still in the gown sleeve and push the opposite (dominant) hand into the glove, lining up the thumb of the glove with the thumb of the dominant hand. As the hand enters the glove, allow it to come out of the sleeve. If all five fingers are not placed correctly in the glove, wait until both gloves are on to adjust them. Repeat the process for the second glove, and adjust gloves as necessary (see **FIGURE 1-10**).

FIGURE 1-10: Place gloves

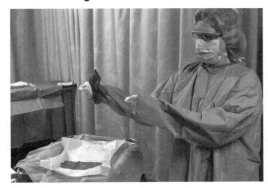

- Gloves that are appropriately donned cover the cuffs of the gown sleeves (see **FIGURE 1-11**). There are three methods for donning sterile gloves: open, closed, and assisted. If the assisted technique is being used, an already sterilely gloved assistant spreads the glove opening apart while the scrubbed person slides his or her hand into it. This method is the safest (has the least chance of contamination) of the three methods and is the preferred way to change gloves in the event of glove contamination during a procedure.[10]

FIGURE 1-11: Place gloves

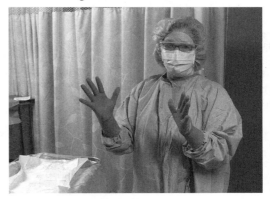

- For clean gloves:
  - Remove a correctly sized pair of gloves from the box and fit them over the fingers and hands, pulling the cuff of the glove over the wrist. Make any finger adjustment as needed.
  - Torn, ripped, or punctured gloves need to be promptly changed.

Step 13: Prepare the Procedure Site

- Skin cleansing for procedures should be done by preparation of a large area (greater than actually required for the procedure) (see **FIGURE 1-12**). The leeway provided by preparation of a large area allows for adjustments in the procedure site, as well as

FIGURE 1-12: Prep skin

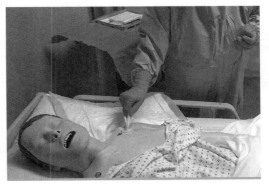

TABLE 1-6: Commonly Used Skin Prep Agents

Agent	Motion	Post-procedure Cleaning	Drying Time
Chlorhexidine gluconate (common brands: Chloraprep, Exidine, Bioscrub, Hibiclens)	Back and forth, going over the area many times	Not required	1–3 minutes, depending on anatomic site
Povidone-iodine solution (common brand: Betadine)	Outward concentric circles,* never going over the same area twice	Required	At least 2 minutes; ensure it is dry
Alcohol (common brand: Alco-prep)	Back and forth, going over the area many times	Not required	1–2 minutes; ensure it is dry

*For indwelling catheter insertion in a female patient, the application of povidone-iodine solution is completed using a top-to-bottom motion, cleaning each section of the insertion area.

the drape if needed, while remaining within an area of sterility. Antimicrobial agent application should be based on the type chosen (see **TABLE 1-6**). Following application of the skin-prep agent, allow time for the agent to fully dry. Do not fan the area, because this may cause contamination of the site.

- Subsequent to the completion of the procedure, any remaining povidone-iodine agent needs to be removed. The easiest way to complete this is to moisten a piece of gauze with sterile saline and gently clean the area. Additionally, if there is blood at the procedure site, regardless of agent used, this too could be cleaned in the same manner.

Step 14: Drape Area

- Many procedures necessitate draping. The types of draping needed for the most commonly performed procedures are delineated in **TABLE 1-7**. Some procedures require full

TABLE 1-7: Draping Requirements for Common Bedside Procedures

Procedure	Drape Type	Below Site Drape
Peripheral IV, routine phlebotomy	None	Clean Chux recommended
Indwelling urinary catheter	Fenestrated optional	Sterile drape (shiny side down) below procedure site required
Central venous catheter	Fenestrated, full-body drape	Clean Chux applied below site prior to donning sterile PPE and prepping the patient
Thoracentesis, paracentesis, lumbar puncture, arterial line, and bone marrow aspiration	Fenestrated, partial drape	Sterile drape (shiny side down) below procedure site required

maximum barrier draping; for these, a large **fenestrated** (a hole in the drape through which the procedure is performed) drape is used. An adhesive area may surround the fenestration and is revealed by removal of the protective paper covering the adhesive. The fenestration is then applied over the intended site of the procedure (the intended procedure site should be in the middle of the opening) and pressed firmly down to facilitate adherence of the drape to the patient's skin. The adhesive area helps to prevent movement of the drape during the procedure and secures the sterile area in which the procedure is to be performed. The drape is then held down with one hand over the sterile site and carefully unfolded over the patient's head and body.

- Other procedures require the use of only a local barrier. These procedures may use a smaller fenestrated drape. The same principles for application are practiced. The protective paper is removed from the fenestrated area, if applicable, and applied over the intended site of the procedure (see **FIGURE 1-13**). Finally, the drape is secured with one hand and unfolded, as indicated earlier.
- Some procedures do not require such draping, but all require the preparation of an area in which the procedure is to be performed.
- Additional drapes may be used to build a larger sterile or clean area. This ensures a continuous field and can serve as an absorptive area for fluids. It is good practice to include placing draping materials that have absorptive qualities below the site of the procedure to catch any body fluids that may drip. Depending on the procedure, these may be clean or sterile.

Step 15: Prepare a Sterile Field

- For many procedures, preparation of a sterile field can be accomplished by draping an area near the patient, although the bed should be avoided for housing the equipment necessary for procedural performance. For most procedures, it is necessary to obtain a bedside table or instrument stand. A sterile drape can be used to prepare the field on which the equipment will be placed. Unless absolutely necessary, drapes overlaid on the patient for use as a working surface should be avoided. For procedures that do not require sterile draping of any kind (routine phlebotomy and peripheral IVs), a clean, dry table with or without a clean drape may be used to hold equipment.

Step 16: Open and Prepare the Kit

- For sterile procedures:
  - Commercial vendors supply kits for most procedures. Becoming familiar with the types of kits used at one's institution facilitates correct sequestration and usage. Kits can be opened with or without the help of an assistant. If an assistant is not available, the outer, non-sterile covering of the kit should be opened prior to performing hand hygiene and donning sterile gloves. Once the provider has donned sterile gloves, any sterile part of the kit may be safely handled. Some kits do not contain all necessary items. Any omitted items obtained elsewhere should be removed from the non-sterile packaging and dropped onto the sterile field or into the kit with the help of an assistant.

FIGURE 1-13: Drape the area

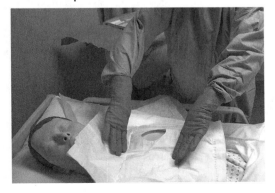

- For clean/semi-sterile procedures (routine phlebotomy and peripheral intravenous catheters):
  - The kits and other equipment can be handled with clean hands or gloves except for the area cleaned on the patient's skin and the needle/catheter end, which will penetrate the skin.

Step 17: If Using Ultrasound, Prepare the Probe

- For procedures requiring the use of ultrasound (e.g., central venous catheter insertion), the probe must be draped with a sterile sleeve prior to use during the procedure. In order to accomplish this, the help of an assistant may be necessary. The assistant will apply non-sterile gel to the transducer head. The assistant will then hold the probe up so that the healthcare provider can grab the probe using the sterile sleeve. The healthcare provider will insert his or her hand into the probe cover, grab the end of the probe from the assistant, and hold firmly onto the probe while the assistant pulls the sleeve completely down, being careful to touch only the edge of the sleeve's end (see **FIGURE 1-14**).
- Rubber bands found in the sleeve package are then applied at the distal end of the probe, around its head (note: avoid rubber bands around the insulated wire connecting the probe to the ultrasound unit) so that the sleeve fits tightly over the end, without

FIGURE 1-14: Prepare the probe

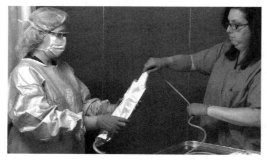

any air between the transducer head and the sleeve. Sterile gel is then applied to the outer surface of the sleeve, to the part that will come in contact with the skin. Once sheathed, the probe may safely and sterilely rest on the sterile field until it is needed.

Step 18: Maintain the Environment

- Once the provider is fully prepared and the sterile field is set, maintenance of the environment is critical:
  - Non-sterile items may not come in contact with any part of the sterile field, the prepped procedure site, or the gloves or gown of the healthcare provider.
  - Nothing below the table, or the provider's waist, is considered sterile. Generally, the front of the gown, from the chest to the level of the sterile field, is considered the sterile window. Sleeves are considered sterile from 2 inches above the elbow to the sleeve cuff. Sleeve cuffs are considered contaminated once the provider's hands pass through them; therefore, if a glove needs to be changed, it should be done with the help of an assistant or by the open glove method. This underscores the importance of ensuring the cuffs are completely inside the sterile gloves.
  - When moving around a sterile area, the front of the healthcare provider is the only area considered sterile and therefore must always face the sterile field. When moving around other persons who are also wearing sterile gowns, passage occurs either front-to-front or back-to-back, never turning one's back directly to the sterile field.
  - Hands must always remain above the waist. While waiting to perform a procedure, and wearing PPE, hands should be clasped together and held above the waist close to the body, never down at one's sides or under the armpits.
  - All persons within the sterile field should don caps, masks, sterile gowns, and

sterile gloves, if applicable to the procedure. Persons within the room, but not in the sterile area, should don hats and masks at a minimum.

- Sterile fields should be prepared as close to the time of the procedure as possible. Time delay between preparation and procedural performance increases the possibility of contamination.

- The sterile working area should be prepared in close proximity to the site of ultimate procedural performance so as to ensure a contiguous sterile field. This is comprised of three aspects: the operator in a sterile gown, the sterile working area, and the sterile site of the planned procedure.

- Conversations by other personnel in the room, who may not be wearing a mask, should be kept to a minimum to reduce the possibility of droplet contamination of a sterile field.

POST-PROCEDURE

Step 19: Clean the Procedural Site and Apply a Sterile Dressing

- Procedural sites should be cleaned with sterile saline and gauze to remove residual skin-prep agents and/or blood. Once the area is clean and dry, a sterile dressing should be applied. Some procedures have specific dressing requirements, thus familiarity with the post-procedure dressing requirements is recommended.

Step 20: Remove and Dispose of the Drapes

- All draping materials should be removed with care taken not to dislodge dressings or medical equipment that has been placed. Soiled drapery, or those contaminated with any bodily fluids, should be disposed of in appropriate biohazard bags and receptacles. Drapes should be folded inward to contain bodily fluids and to avoid any spillage.

Step 21: Dispose of Sharps

- With gloves still on, all sharps should be carefully located and disposed of in the appropriate sharps container. Ensure that all sharps are indeed removed before discarding the rest of the kit and/or equipment in the biohazard receptacle.

Step 22: Discard PPE

- All PPE needs to be removed, discarded, and placed in an appropriate biohazard receptacle. Generally, the exterior gown, sleeves, and any visibly soiled surfaces are considered contaminated, so these areas should not be handled with bare hands during the removal process. Clean areas are the inside of the gloves, interior and back of the gown including the ties, and the ties of the mask; the goggles and face shield are also considered clean. Clean areas can safely be handled during the removal process. PPE should be removed in close proximity to the container in which it will be discarded.

- Gloves should be removed first, taking care to avoid touching the outer part of the gloves with bare hands. Grasp the outside edge of the cuff of the glove and peel the glove off while turning it inside out. Hold the glove in the opposite hand, and slide two fingers inside the remaining glove, touching only the inside of the glove while peeling off the glove, turning it inside out so that the first glove remains inside the second one. Next, remove the gown. Unfasten the ties at the neck and waist, peel the gown away from the neck and shoulders, turning the outside of the gown inward to contain contaminants. Fold or roll the gown into a bundle with the inside of the gown facing outward. Alternatively, the gloves can be removed as a component of gown removal as described earlier. Lastly, remove the hat, mask, and goggles or face shield.

Step 23: Wash Hands

- The final step in aseptic technique is to carry out hand hygiene. An appropriate antiseptic soap or alcohol-based hand rub should be chosen. Appropriate post-procedure handwashing with soap and water should include scrubbing of all surfaces for at least 15–20 seconds, allowing dirty water to run away from clean surfaces, and completely drying with clean disposable towels in a patting motion. If a sink is unavailable, proper hand sanitizing with an alcohol-based hand rub is an alternative to soap and water, provided there is no visible soiling of the hands. This consists of scrubbing all surfaces for at least 15–20 seconds and allowing the agent to dry.

Managing a Break in Sterility

- Any break in sterility leaves the patient and/or the provider susceptible to infection; therefore, impeccable monitoring must occur. Any breaks in sterility must be corrected as soon as they are noted, without second-guessing, debate, or hesitation.
- During procedure setup, all packaging, PPE, and sterile equipment should be examined, looking for intact seals; rips, tears, and expiration dates should also be noted. If any aspect is compromised, those items must be replaced.
- During preparation for and during the performance of the procedure, all providers should monitor for contamination of the sterile field and medical equipment. If any item becomes contaminated at any time, that item needs to be replaced. If previously prepped skin or scrubbed hands become contaminated, prep and/or hand hygiene need to be repeated.
- Items that fall on the floor should be replaced with new items. Gloves that are ripped, torn, or punctured must be replaced. If a healthcare provider encounters a needlestick or any break in the integrity of their own skin, the procedure should be safely stopped, their injury assessed, and institutional policy followed.
- Should it become necessary for a new person to step in during a procedure, the area and sterile field should be completely covered with a sterile drape while the new person performs hand hygiene and dons appropriate PPE. If a second person is not readily available, a completely new setup and prep should be completed.

► REFERENCES

1. Klevens RM, Edwards JR, Richards CL Jr, et al. Estimating health care-associated infections and deaths in U.S. hospitals, 2002. *Public Health Rep.* 2007;122(2):160–166.
2. Office of Disease Prevention and Health Promotion. National Action Plan to Prevent Health Care-Associated Infections: Roadmap to Elimination. http://www.health.gov/hcq/pdfs/hai-action-plan-executive-summary.pdf. Accessed April 17, 2012.
3. Hales B, Pronovost P. The checklist—a tool for error management and performance improvement. *J Crit Care.* 2006;21(3):231–235.
4. Regional Allied Health and Science Initiative. Medical Anatomy and Physiology Curriculum 2010. http://www.haspi.org/curriculum-library/A-P-summaries/Med-A-P-Curriculum-2010.pdf. Accessed April 24, 2012.
5. U.S. Department of Labor. Personal Protective Equipment: OSHA 3151-12R 2003. https://www.osha.gov/Publications/osha3151.pdf. Accessed June 25, 2015.
6. Pellowe C, Loveday H, Pratt R, et al. Standard principles: personal protective equipment and the safe use and disposal of sharps. *Nursing Times.* November 20, 2007. http://www.nursingtimes.net/nursing-practice/specialisms/management/standard-principles-personal-protective-equipment-and-the-safe-use-and-disposal-of-sharps/291502.article. Accessed June 25, 2015.
7. Chalykunapruk N, Veenstra D, Lipsky B, et al. Chlorhexidine compared with povidone-iodine solution for vascular catheter-site care: a meta-analysis. *Ann Intern Med.* 2002;136:79–801.
8. Boyce J, Pittet D. CDC Guideline for Hand Hygiene in Health-Care Settings. Recommendations of the Healthcare Infection control Practices Advisory Committee and the HICPAC/SHEA/APIC/IDSA Hand Hygiene Task Force. *MMWR Recomm Rep.* 2002:51(RR-16):1–45. http://www.cdc.gov/mmwr/preview/mmwrhtml/rr5116a1.htm. Accessed June 25, 2015.
9. Larson E. APIC guideline for hand washing and hand antisepsis in healthcare settings. *Am J Infect Control.* 1995;23:251–69.
10. Hopper W, Moss R. Common breaks in sterile technique: clinical perspectives and perioperative implications. *AORN J.* 2010;19(3);350–367.

► ENDNOTES

i. Throughout the chapter when the term *asepsis* is used, it is understood to mean "general asepsis."
ii. Chlorhexidine gluconate is a cationic bis-biguanide developed in England in the early 1950s and was introduced in the United States in the 1970s. The antimicrobial activity of chlorhexidine is likely attributable to its attachment to, and subsequent disruption of, cytoplasmic membranes, resulting in precipitation of cellular contents.[8]

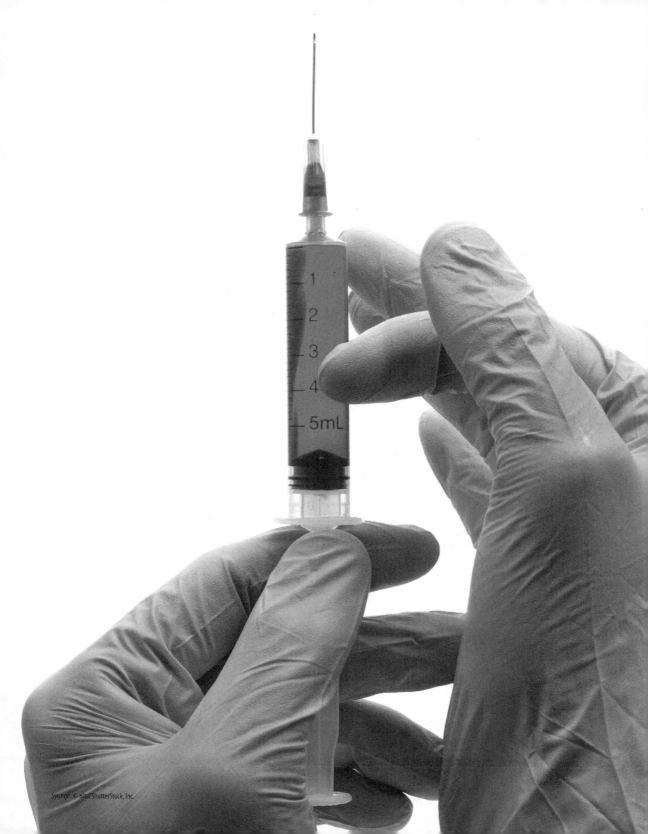

CHAPTER 2

Nasogastric Tube Placement

Linda Wilson, RN, PhD, CPAN, CAPA, BC, CNE, CHSE, CHSE-A, ANEF, FAAN

John Cornele, MSN, RN, CNE, EMT-P

GOALS

▶ Suction stomach contents.

▶ Administer medications and food.

OBJECTIVES

1. Identify and describe common complications associated with performing nasogastric (NG) tube placement.
2. Describe the essential anatomy and physiology associated with the performance of NG tube placement.
3. Identify the materials necessary for performing NG tube placement and their proper use.
4. Describe the steps for correctly inserting an NG tube.
5. Discuss aspects of post-NG tube placement care and follow-up.

RATIONALE

The NG tube is used:

- To drain the stomach pre- or post-surgery
- To lavage the stomach and, with the use of suction, to remove gastric secretions or gas buildups—particularly useful when a patient has decreased or absent peristalsis[1]

EVIDENCE-BASED INDICATIONS

For the insertion of an NG tube, indications include:

- Sampling gastric contents
- Removing air, blood, ingested substances, and gastric contents
- Providing nutritional support for patients who cannot eat but have a functional gastrointestinal (GI) tract

CONTRAINDICATIONS

NG tube placement is contraindicated when the intended path of the tube is obstructed or any of the structures the NG tube would traverse are damaged, as well as in the following situations or conditions:

- **Choanal atresia**
- Significant facial trauma or basilar skull fracture
- **Esophageal stricture** or atresia
- Esophageal burn
- **Zenker diverticulum**
- Recent surgery on the esophagus or stomach
- Sampling gastric contents

COMPLICATIONS

- Aspiration
- Trauma to the turbinates and/or nasopharynx
- Pneumonia caused by tube misplacement

Proper insertion techniques, gentle pressure during tube passage, and patient cooperation will help prevent these problems.

SPECIAL CONSIDERATIONS

- Make sure that the tube has not passed through the larynx and trachea to the bronchi (stethoscope, chest X-ray).

SUPPLIES

Before the procedure, gather the needed equipment:

- NG tube
- General surgical lubrication jelly
- Adhesive tape
- Safety pin
- A 60-mL catheter-tipped irrigation syringe
- Glass of drinking water with a straw
- Tissues
- pH strip and suction equipment

PROCEDURAL INSTRUCTIONS

- Introduce yourself to your patient and explain the procedure. The patient's cooperation helps the procedure go smoothly.
- Put on gloves.
- Place an awake or conscious patient in a sitting position.
- Approximate the length of the NG tube to be inserted by measuring the distance from the nares to the stomach (see **FIGURE 2-1**). This is done by placing the tip of the NG tube at

FIGURE 2-1: Approximate NG tube length

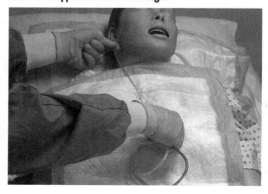

the patient's nose and extending the tube via the earlobe to the tip of the xyphoid process.[2]

- Mark the NG tube with a piece of tape where it reaches the xyphoid process. The purpose of the tape is to mark the NG tube at the point where it will reach the correct location in the patient's stomach.[2]
- To determine which nasal passage is the clearest, and will therefore enable the smoothest insertion of the NG tube, gently press your finger to the outside of one of the patient's nostrils and listen to the patient breathe through the open nostril. Repeat the process with the other nostril and compare the results (see **FIGURE 2-2**).
- Lubricate the first 4 inches of the NG tube with surgical lubrication jelly.
- If the patient is unconscious, place the patient in a supine position for the procedure and use a water-soluble lubricant.
- If someone is available to assist with the procedure, have the assistant hold the patient's head forward gently or ask the patient to do this (see **FIGURE 2-3**). This position will open up the esophagus and slightly close the trachea. Later during the insertion—when you ask the patient to swallow—the trachea will close off further.
- Begin insertion of the NG tube into the predetermined nostril. After reaching the hypopharynx, pause slightly to allow the patient to adjust to the feel of the NG tube.

FIGURE 2-2: Identify nostril patency

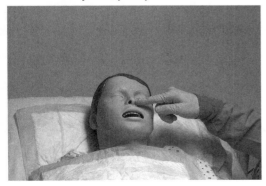

FIGURE 2-3: Tilt the head

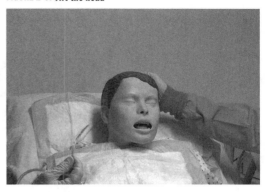

FIGURE 2-4: Advance the tube

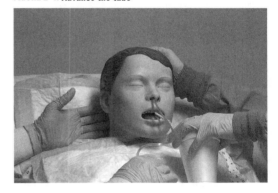

- Then, have the patient swallow each time the NG tube is advanced until the tube has been inserted up to the initial marker on the tube (see **FIGURE 2-4**).
- If the patient's eyes tear up during the insertion, gently dab the patient's eyes with a tissue or offer it to him or her.
- Before securing the tube, take a sample of the drainage using the syringe to make sure the tube has been inserted into the correct location (see **FIGURE 2-5**).
- After drawing a sample of gastric contents and confirming the placement of the tube, secure the tube with a piece of tape to the patient's nose.
- It is helpful to tear the tape before the procedure into three tails approximately 3 inches in length.

FIGURE 2-5: Obtain sample

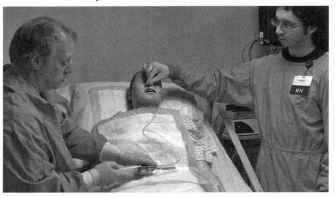

FIGURE 2-6: Use tape to fix NG tube

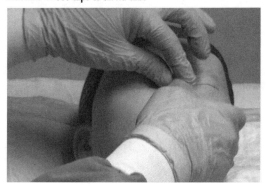

FIGURE 2-7: Secure the tube

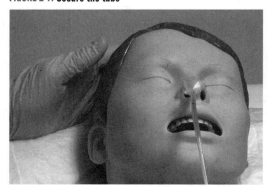

- Place the non-torn base of the tape on the patient's nose (see **FIGURE 2-6**).
- Affix the middle tail down the length of the NG tube and wrap the other two tails on either side around the tube in opposite directions to prevent tube migration (see **FIGURE 2-7**).
- Farther down the tube, around the area of the patient's chest, wrap a piece of tape around the NG tube, leaving excess tape sticking out, and stick a safety pin through the excess tape to attach the tube to the patient's gown. This securing of the NG tube will prevent the NG tube from becoming dislodged or repositioned and will also prevent patient discomfort.
- Once the NG tube is in place and secured, aspirate gastric contents into the 60-mL

syringe, and then test the aspirate for acidity using the pH strips (see **FIGURE 2-8**). The blue litmus paper should turn red immediately.

FIGURE 2-8: Test sample

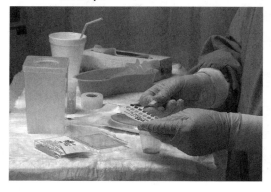

- If you are not able to aspirate gastric contents, fill the 60-mL syringe with air and reconnect it to the NG tube. Make sure to close off the air vent (blue pigtail) prior to injecting the air. Inject the air through the main lumen of the NG tube and auscultate over the stomach while injecting the air.[2]
- If the NG tube is correctly positioned, there will be an obvious, audible gurgling noise auscultated over the stomach.

AFTERCARE INSTRUCTIONS

- After the procedure, check the patient's chart to see if there is an order for an X-ray to verify tube placement.
- Once the placement of the NG tube has been verified, connect the NG tube to suction.
- The drainage from the NG tube should be emptied, measured, and documented.

► REFERENCES

1. Ellis JR, Bentz PM. *Modules for Basic Nursing Skills.* 7th ed. Philadelphia: Lippincott Williams & Wilkins; 2007.
2. Baskett PJ, Dow A, Nolan J, et al. *Practical Procedures in Anesthesia and Critical Care.* London: Mosby; 1995.

► ADDITIONAL READING

Perry AG, Potter P. *Clinical Nursing Skills and Techniques.* 6th ed. Philadelphia: Elsevier Mosby; 2006.

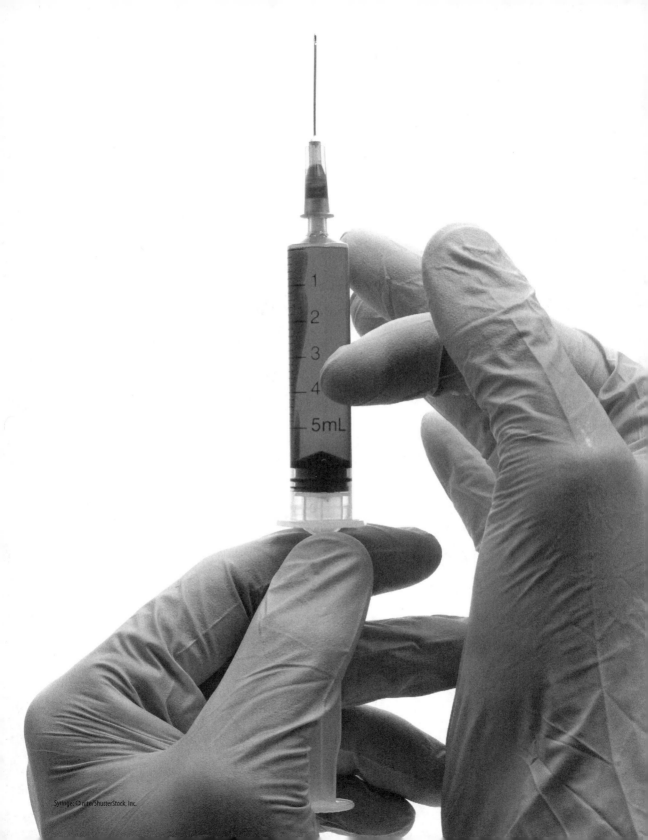

CHAPTER 3

Urinary Catheterization

Carol Okupniak, DNP, RN-BC

GOALS

▶ Understand the rationale for draining the urinary **bladder** using a urinary **catheter**.

▶ Understand the steps involved in **urinary catheterization** for single use or continuous drainage.

▶ Recognize that urinary catheters are made from a variety of materials.

▶ Understand catheter measurements: The size of the catheter is measured in French units (Fr or F). A **French** unit is equivalent to 0.33 millimeters or 0.013 inches. Catheters range in size from 3.5 to 30 Fr, with the most common sizes for adults from 12 to 18 Fr.

OBJECTIVES

1. Demonstrate the knowledge and ability to perform urinary catheterization.
2. Understand potential complications of urinary catheterization.
3. Demonstrate knowledge of contraindications and complications of urinary catheterization.

RATIONALE

- **Urine** output monitoring
  - Patients with low cardiac output or impaired renal function often require urinary catheterization to accurately monitor urine output.
- Chronically bedridden patients
  - Patients who are bedridden are candidates for urinary catheterization. Examples include patients with spinal cord injuries, unconscious patients, and patients with urinary incontinence.

TYPES OF URINARY CATHETERS

- **Foley catheters** come in several models. A commonly used subtype is the "triple-lumen" or "three-way" catheter (see **TABLE 3-1**). The triple lumen has a primary channel with openings at each end to drain urine, a secondary channel with a balloon near the tip that is inflated with sterile water to keep the catheter in place, and a third channel that is used to instill irrigation solution.
- Details on other catheters such as the **non-retention catheter**, **Robinson catheter**, **silastic catheter**, **silicone catheter**, and **three-way catheter** are in Table 3-1.
- Another subtype of Foley is the **Coudé-tipped catheter** (see Table 3-1), with models called the **Tiemann catheter** and the **Carson catheter**. The Coudé has a 45° angle at the tip that helps when inserted over an enlarged prostate or navigating the neck of the bladder in female patients.
- Another type, the "Councill tip" has a reinforced hole at the tip through which a **Councill tip stylet** can be passed. This type can be used to open the urethra in emergency situations when a stricture or enlarged prostate block restricts urine flow until a surgical intervention can be completed.

EVIDENCE-BASED INDICATIONS

Urinary catheters are used in the following situations:

- Acute **urinary retention**
- Urethral surgery
- Abdominal or genitourinary surgery to decompress the bladder prior to incision
- Anesthetized or sedated patients undergoing surgery
- Comatose or semi-comatose patients
- Incontinence
- Paralysis
- Physical injury when unable to use toilet facilities or urinals
- Enlarged prostate when urine flow is blocked
- Medical conditions that block or limit urine flow, such as uterine fibroid tumors in women
- Need for precise measurement of urine output

CONTRAINDICATIONS

- The main contraindication for urethral catheterization is suspected urethral injury following pelvic trauma.
- Blood at the urethral meatus, bruising to the scrotum, and significant mechanism of trauma involving the pelvic region are indications to withhold catheterization until the patient is assessed further.
- Acute urethral and prostate infection.
- Urinary catheterization is cautioned in patients with suspected acute myocardial infarction.

COMPLICATIONS

Infection

- The insertion of a urinary catheter provides a direct route for bacteria to enter the urinary tract. Handwashing, proper preparation of the site, and adherence to aseptic technique are critical to reduce this complication.

TABLE 3-1: Types of Urinary Catheters

Catheter Type	Characteristics	Uses
Non-retention catheter (e.g., Robinson catheter, straight catheter)	• **Straight catheter** • Lumen at tip and end for drainage	• Obtain sterile urine specimen • Relieve postoperative urine retention • Measure residual urine
Retention catheter (e.g., Foley catheter)	• Designed to remain in the bladder for extended periods • Drainage lumen—for urine outflow • Inflation lumen for balloon—a channel in the tube allows for insertion of water into a balloon (once the catheter is inserted) to prevent the catheter from slipping out of bladder into urethra Size range: 3.5–30 Fr Adult male: 16–20 Fr Balloon sizes: 5- to 30-mL capacity No need to inflate the balloon to 30-mL capacity if only using for urine drainage	• Continuous drainage for accurate intake and output monitoring • Postoperative care of patient to allow area to heal • Keep incontinent patient dry
Three-way catheter (e.g., Foley catheter)	Designed to remain in bladder for irrigation Three ports: 1. Tube for urine drainage 2. Tube for inflation of balloon 3. Tube for instillation of irrigation fluid Larger size range of catheters (30-mL inflate) is required for continuous irrigation to allow for drainage of clots, mucous, and sediment. Balloon must be inflated to maximum capacity for irrigation.	Continuous bladder irrigation following prostate/genitourinary surgery, to maintain catheter patency—removes small blood clots and mucous Closed system to reduce introduction of pathogens Traction frequently applied to catheter
Coudé catheter	Curved, rounded rigid tip	Easier to insert in the male urethra when the prostate is enlarged
Silicone catheter	Similar to a Foley, except more rigid Only latex-free catheter	*Latex allergy*
Silastic catheter	Usually green color Can stay in for extended period of time	Can stay in 3–6 months

- Urinary tract infection is a major problem associated with **indwelling catheters**. This is due to bacteria traveling up the catheter to the bladder. Some manufacturers provide catheters that have been coated with antiseptic to help combat this problem.
- With long-term use, a catheter can become coated with biofilm. This biofilm can obstruct drainage, resulting in stagnant urine left in the bladder contributing to urinary tract infections.

Trauma

- Inserting a urinary catheter can cause trauma to the urethra.
- If the catheter is lubricated with sterile, water-soluble lubricant, this reduces the incidence of trauma to the urethral canal and eases insertion.
- Never force the catheter against resistance. If resistance is felt, ask the patient to bear down as if to void. This may allow further advancement of the catheter.

Restricted Canal

- Urethral stricture or an enlarged prostate gland can reduce the diameter of the urethra. If the patient has a known or suspected history of this, consider using a smaller catheter.

Vaginal Catheterization

- Inadvertent catheterization of the vaginal canal is a complication of urinary catheterization. This will manifest as the absence of urine return despite ease of insertion.
- Proper patient positioning can reduce the incidence of this occurring.
- If vaginal catheterization is suspected, remove the catheter and discard it, because it is now contaminated. Reattempt urinary catheterization with a new catheter. (Note: Some healthcare providers will leave this catheter in place to aid in locating the urethral meatus prior to the next attempt.)

Inability to Locate Urethra

- The incidence of the inability to locate the urethra in female patients can be reduced by proper preparation. Correct patient positioning and thorough cleansing of the periurethral area will assist in locating the urethra and surrounding anatomic landmarks.

Supply Complications

- *Balloon breakage during catheter insertion.* A healthcare provider must remove balloon fragments.
- *Balloon not inflating after insertion.* Some institutional protocols require that the balloon be tested prior to insertion. If the balloon does not inflate, the catheter should be removed and a new catheter placed.
- *Urine flow stoppage.* Provider checks for positioning or obstruction in the tube. If obstructed, an attempt can be made to flush the catheter with sterile saline. If the blockage cannot be relieved, the catheter is removed and discarded.
- *Opening the balloon prior to complete insertion of the catheter into the bladder.* This error can result in urethral damage.
- *Defective catheters, which break in situ.* This problem usually occurs near the balloon or at the tip.
- *Leaking tube or drainage system.* If the system is damaged, it will have to be removed and replaced.
- *Patient pulls catheter out.* This can result in severe injury and may require emergency treatment.

SUPPLIES

- Sterile urinary catheterization kit:
  - Gloves
  - Drapes
  - Lubricant
  - Antiseptic cleaning solution
  - Cotton balls
  - Forceps
  - Prefilled syringe with sterile water used to inflate balloon after insertion (check balloon function prior to insertion if required by institutional policy)
  - Catheter (intermittent or indwelling)

- Sterile drainage tubing and collection bag if indwelling
- Receptacle or basin for collecting urine if intermittent
- Specimen container
- Sheet to drape for patient
- Waterproof absorbent pad under the buttocks and perineum
- Disposable gloves
- Basin with warm water, soap, washcloth, and towel
- Light source

PROCEDURAL INSTRUCTIONS

General Assessment

- Review the medical record and identify the purpose of inserting a catheter.
- Will the patient require irrigation of the catheter after insertion?
- Will a sterile urine specimen be collected?
- Will residual urine be measured?
- Has the patient had a urinary catheterization in the past?
- If the patient has been catheterized, what was the prior response to catheterization?
- If catheterized previously, when was the last catheterization?
- Determine the type and size of urinary catheter you will use.
  - For adults, most institutions routinely use size 16 Fr catheters. If a 16 Fr is leaking around the urethra, an 18 Fr catheter can be used. If it is difficult to insert a 14 Fr catheter due to a narrow urethra or medical condition causing narrowing of the urethra, a 12 Fr catheter can be used.
  - For children, follow institutional policy.
- Determine if institutional policy limits maximum amount of urine drained with each catheterization (800–1000 mL).

Assess the Patient

- Determine the time of the patient's last urination.

- What is the patient's level of consciousness, developmental stage, and awareness of the procedure?
- Are there any mobility or physical limitations?
- Verify gender and age.
- Assess the bladder for distention.
- Assess for erythema, drainage from the urethra, or odor.
- Identify any pathology that may interfere with passage of the catheter.
- Assess the patient's knowledge and purpose for urinary catheterization.
- Assess for anatomic landmarks and visualize urethral opening.
- Determine allergy:
  - Antiseptic—if povidone-iodine solution (Betadine) is part of the catheter kit and the patient is unaware of allergy, ask if allergic to shellfish.

Expected Outcomes

- Patient understands the procedure.
- Bladder is not palpable after urine is drained through catheter.
- Patient verbalizes relief of discomfort and minimal pain or discomfort during procedure.
- A minimum of 30 milliliters of urine is present hourly in the collection bag if indwelling (adult patient).

Prepare for Urinary Catheter Insertion[1]

- Provide for privacy.
- Raise the bed to appropriate working height.
- Perform hand hygiene.
- If right-handed, stand on the left side of bed; stand on the right side if left-handed.
- Ensure side rail is raised on opposite side and lowered on working side.
- Place waterproof pad under patient's buttocks and perineum.
- Place patient in proper position for urinary catheterization:
  - Female:
    - Dorsal recumbent (supine with knees flexed).

FIGURE 3-1: Prepare supplies

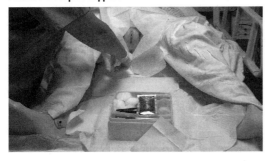

- ◆ Ask patient to relax thighs, which will externally rotate the hips.
- ◆ If unable to assume supine position, ask patient to assume Sims, or side-lying, position with upper leg flexed at hip and knee (cover rectal area with drape to reduce risk of cross-contamination).
- ▪ Male:
  - ◆ Supine with thighs slightly abducted
- Drape patient (see **FIGURE 3-1**):
  - ▪ Female—use blanket with one corner at head, two over arms, last corner covering legs and over perineum, then lift and fold last corner so that genitalia is exposed.
  - ▪ Male—cover upper trunk with sheet or blanket, with lower extremities covered, leaving only genitalia exposed.
- Wearing disposable, non-sterile gloves, cleanse perineal area with soap and warm water and dry with towel.
- Position light source to illuminate perineal area.
- Perform hand hygiene.
- Open urinary catheterization kit according to package directions, keeping the bottom of kit sterile.
- Use bag the kit comes in for disposal and keep close to sterile field without contamination.
- If waterproof underpad is the first item in the kit, carefully place plastic side down under the patient, touching only the edges and maintaining sterility.
- Apply sterile gloves.

- Organize supplies on the sterile field:
  - ▪ Open inner sterile package.
  - ▪ Pour antiseptic solution into compartment with cotton balls.
  - ▪ Open lubricant package or remove cap from syringe containing lubrication and fill compartment with lubricant.
  - ▪ Remove specimen container, ensuring lid is loosely placed on top, and place aside on sterile field.
  - ▪ Remove prefilled syringe used to inflate balloon if indwelling catheter and place aside on sterile field.
  - ▪ Follow manufacturer's recommendations or institutional policy: Inject sterile fluid from prefilled syringe into balloon port to ensure integrity of balloon. If performing this step, deflate the balloon completely, removing syringe from the balloon port, and ensure that catheter remains within the sterile field (see **FIGURE 3-2**). There is some discussion that this step is unnecessary and may stretch the balloon, causing trauma on insertion.
- Lubricate catheter tip (if plastic sheath, remove before lubricating):
  - ▪ Female—2.5 to 5 cm (1 to 2 inches)
  - ▪ Male—12.5 to 17.5 cm (5 to 7 inches)
- Apply sterile drape, keeping gloves sterile:
  - ▪ Female
    - ◆ Top edge of drape to form cuff over sterile gloves.
    - ◆ Place drape between thighs.

FIGURE 3-2: Test catheter for leaks

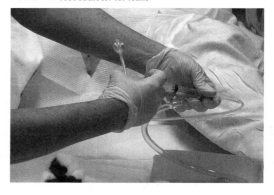

- Slip cuffed edge just under buttocks, making sure to not contaminate sterile gloves.
- Unfold fenestrated drape without touching unsterile objects.
- Apply drape over perineum, exposing labia without contaminating sterile gloves.
  - Male (two methods)
    - (1) Apply drape over thighs and below penis without opening.
    - (2) Apply folded drape over thighs just below penis, pick up edge, allowing to unfold, and drape over penis with fenestration over penis.
- Place sterile tray and contents on sterile drape.
- Cleanse urethral meatus (see **FIGURE 3-3**):
  - Female
    - With nondominant hand, retract labia to expose urethral meatus (maintain position of nondominant hand during remaining procedure). If labia release during cleaning, retract labia again and repeat cleansing procedure.
    - With dominant hand, use forceps to pick up antiseptic-coated cotton ball and use it to wipe perineal area from front to back (clitoris to anus) using a new cotton ball for each area, starting at labia majora, then labia minora, and finally over the center

FIGURE 3-3: Cleanse periurethral area

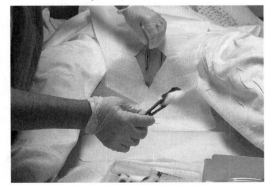

of urethral meatus; dispose of each cotton ball after single use.
  - Male
    - Uncircumcised—with nondominant hand, grasp penis at shaft just below glans and retract foreskin between thumb and forefinger (maintain position of nondominant hand during remaining procedure). If foreskin released during cleaning, retract foreskin again and repeat cleansing procedure.
    - Circumcised and uncircumcised—with dominant hand, use forceps to pick up cotton ball; starting at urethral meatus move cotton ball in a circular motion from the urethra to the base of the glans; repeat cleansing three more times using a new cotton ball each time.
- With dominant hand, grasp catheter 7.5 to 10 cm (3 to 4 inches) from top; hold end loosely coiled in palm of hand (if straight or single-use catheter, make sure open or distal end of catheter is placed in urine receptacle).

Insert Catheter

- Female
  - Ask patient to gently bear down as if to urinate and slowly insert catheter through urethral meatus 5 to 7.5 cm (2 to 3 inches) in adult or until urine flows; as soon as urine appears, advance an additional 5 to 7.5 cm (2 to 3 inches) without forcing (if no urine appears, it may be in the vagina; if in vagina, leave in place and begin procedure again with a new, sterile catheter).
  - With nondominant hand, remove thumb and forefinger from labia and hold catheter securely.
- Male
  - With nondominant hand, hold penis at a 90° angle to patient's body and apply slight traction, straightening urethral canal during insertion.

- Ask patient to gently bear down as if to urinate and slowly insert catheter through urethral meatus 17 to 22.5 cm (7 to 9 inches) in adult or until urine flows; if resistance is felt, withdraw, do not force; when urine flows, advance to the bifurcation at the catheter distal end and balloon port.
  - With nondominant hand, lower penis and release, and hold catheter securely near distal end.
  - If uncircumcised, reposition foreskin.
- For straight or single-use catheters:
  - If urine specimen collection is required, allow a small amount of urine to flow into collection container before filling specimen cup to desired level (20–30 mL) and carefully put aside; continue to hold distal end of catheter in dominant hand over urine-collection container.
- Determine if institutional policy limits maximum amount of urine drained with each catheterization (500–1000 mL).
- Allow bladder to empty completely unless institutional policy restricts maximum volume.

Straight, Single-Use Catheter Removal

- Ensure that absorbent drape or pad is under the penis (male) or perineum (female) before withdrawal.
- Perform hand hygiene and wear non-sterile gloves.
- Remove catheter with a slow, continuous, steady motion until completely withdrawn from urethra.
- Wrap catheter in absorbent pad.
- Carefully remove urine-collection container to area for measurement and disposal.
- Dispose of all material.
- Remove gloves.
- Ensure that side rails are raised and bed is in a low position.
- Perform hand hygiene and wear non-sterile gloves.
- Clean and dry perineum (female) or glans (male).

- Cover patient's genitalia and assist patient to a position of comfort.
- Placing urine-collection container on a flat, level surface, measure amount, note color and consistency of urine, and dispose of urine into proper receptacle.
- Remove gloves and perform hand hygiene.

Complete Indwelling Catheter Procedure

- To anchor catheter in place above bladder outlet and prevent removal, the balloon must be inflated:
  - With nondominant hand, hold the distal end of the catheter near bifurcation.
  - With dominant hand, attach fluid-filled syringe to balloon port.
  - Very slowly inject all of the solution (if patient experiences pain, remove all solution and advance catheter and attempt to inflate balloon again).
  - After inflating balloon with all fluid, remove syringe and release catheter.
  - Gently pull on catheter to ensure balloon is inflated and holds catheter securely in the bladder.
  - After assessing balloon inflation, advance catheter slightly back into bladder.
- If not preconnected, attach distal end of catheter to the clear tubing of the drainage system.
- Maintain drainage bag below the level of the bladder (do not place on side rails of bed).
- Anchor drainage bag (see **FIGURE 3-4**):
  - Female—secure tubing to inner thigh with nonallergenic tape or an elastic tube holder with Velcro closure; leave enough tubing so there is no tension on the catheter.
  - Male—secure tubing to top of thigh with nonallergenic tape or an elastic tube holder with Velcro closure; catheter can be attached to lower abdomen (penis directed toward chest) with nonallergenic tape; leave enough tubing so there is no tension on the catheter.

FIGURE 3-4: Attach catheter to patient leg

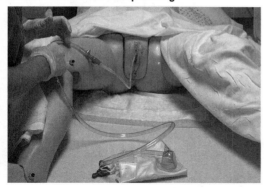

- Ensure tubing is not kinked or obstructed; twist excessive tubing and attach to sheet with clip from kit or with rubber band and safety pin.
- Assist patient to assume a position of comfort.
- Wash and dry perineal area (female) or glans (male).
- Remove gloves, and remove and dispose of all equipment.
- If urine collected, record amount and send to laboratory if ordered, or dispose of urine in proper receptacle.

Evaluation

- Palpate bladder—distention should be relieved.
- Assess patient's level of comfort.
- Observe amount, color, and consistency of urine in drainage system if indwelling catheter.
- Ensure that no urine is leaking from the continuous drainage system.
- Observe amount, color, and consistency of urine in urine-collection container if straight or intermittent catheterization.

Documenting Procedure

- Indicate the reason for urinary catheterization.
- Document the type and size of catheter used.

- Record the amount of fluid inserted into the balloon.
- Document the amount of urine, its color, and consistency.
- If specimens collected, note the date, time the specimen was sent to the laboratory, and the specific test ordered.
- Record the patient's response to the procedure.

Care of Indwelling Catheter[1,2]

- Catheter care
  - Every 8 hours the perineum and first 4 inches of the urinary catheter should be cleaned with mild soap and water.
  - Secretions or encrustations at the catheter insertion site must be removed by gently loosening with mild soap and a wet cloth.
  - Powders or lotions should not be used due to the risk of microbial growth.
- Measuring amount of urine
  - Empty urine drainage bag per institutional policy, when bag is near full, or at least every 8 hours.
  - Using a graduated cylinder, open drainage port on urine-collection bag and drain urine.
  - Empty drainage bag completely or to highest measurable level on graduated cylinder.
  - Place graduated cylinder on a flat surface where it can be viewed at eye level.
  - Visualize and note amount of urine in graduated cylinder.
  - Empty any additional urine from drainage bag following the same procedure.
  - Record total amount of urine in patient's output record.
  - Note color, consistency, and any odor of urine.

Removal of Indwelling Catheter

- Planning
  - Determine how long indwelling urinary catheter has been in place.

- Discontinue or change urinary catheter according to institutional policy or when given an order to discontinue.
- Observe if there is any discharge or encrustations around the catheter insertion site.
- Assess the patient for complaints of pain and determine location, type, and quality of pain.
- Monitor patient's intake and output.
- Assess urine color, consistency, amount, and odor.
- Inform patient of removal procedure.
- Outcomes
  - No secretions or encrustations are present.
  - Urine is clear with adequate volume.
  - Patient is afebrile.
  - Patient has no complaints of pain during removal procedure.
  - After removal, patient voids without discomfort in adequate amounts within 6 to 8 hours of catheter removal.

Removal

- Gather equipment
  - Soap, water, basin, washcloth
  - Non-sterile gloves
  - Graduated cylinder
  - Syringe of adequate size to remove fluid from balloon
  - Waterproof pad
- Perform hand hygiene; apply non-sterile gloves.
- Provide for privacy.
- Raise bed to appropriate working height.
- Place waterproof pad between thighs (female) or over thighs (male).
- Obtain sterile specimen if indicated.
- Remove tape or Velcro strap.
- Insert syringe into balloon port.
- Remove entire amount of fluid used to inflate balloon.
- Pull catheter out with a slow, continuous, steady motion.
- Wrap catheter in waterproof pad.
- Remove drainage bag from bed.

- When catheter removal is completed:
  - Reposition patient and ensure safety by raising side rails and lowering bed if indicated.
  - Empty contents of drainage bag and note amount, color, consistency, and odor. Dispose of all contaminated equipment.
  - Remove gloves and perform hand hygiene.
- Cleansing and skin assessment
  - Perform hand hygiene.
  - Raise bed to working height.
  - Apply non-sterile gloves.
  - Place absorbent pad under buttocks (female) or over thighs (male).
  - Assess skin around urethral opening.
  - Cleans the patient's perineum (female) or glans (male).
  - Remove any remaining tape or adhesive residue from skin; assess skin under adhesive or around tube holder.
  - Lower patient's bed and ensure side rails are raised and secure if indicated.
  - Dispose of gloves and perform hand hygiene.

Documenting Removal

- Document date and time catheter was removed.
- Note character and amount of final urine in drainage bag.
- Observe and record condition of urethral meatus.
- Note condition of skin where adhesive or tube holder was placed.
- Document the time when patient is due to void, usually 6 to 8 hours after catheter removal.

SPECIAL CONSIDERATIONS

Pediatric considerations in urinary catheterization:
- Ensure the child has been given an age-appropriate explanation of the procedure.
- Ensure that the parent(s) or legal guardian has been given an explanation of the purpose and need for urinary catheterization.

- Determine if the child has any genitourinary congenital anomalies that may interfere with urinary catheterization.
- Determine catheter size (these sizes are approximate guides). Always use the smallest catheter size for the child's comfort that will provide adequate drainage:
  - 6 Fr up to 2 years of age
  - 8 Fr for 2–10 years of age
  - 10 Fr for 10–14 years of age
  - 12 Fr for 14 years and older
- Using a lubricant with 2% lidocaine may help ease insertion in infants or young children.

► **REFERENCES**

1. Lynn PB. *Taylor's Clinical Nursing Skills: A Nursing Process Approach.* 3rd ed. Baltimore: Wolters Kluwer Health/Lippincott Williams & Wilkins; 2011:616–635.
2. Nettina S, Ed. *The Lippincott Manual of Nursing Practice.* Ambler, PA: Wolters Kluwer Health/Lippincott Williams & Wilkins, 10th ed.; 2014:777–783.

► **ADDITIONAL READING**

Hooton TM. (2015). Nosocomial urinary tract infections. In: Bennett J, Dolin R, Blaser MJ, eds. *Mandell, Douglas, and Bennett's Principles and Practice of Infectious Diseases.* 8th ed. Philadelphia: Elsevier Saunders.

James RE, Fowler GC. Bladder catheterization (and urethral dilation). In: Albihai H, Broomfield J, Esherick J, et al., eds. *Pfenninger and Fowler's Procedures for Primary Care.* 3rd ed. Philadelphia: Mosby; 2011: 765–769.

Nicolle LE. Urinary catheter-associated infections. *Infect Dis Clin North Am.* 2012;26(1):13–27.

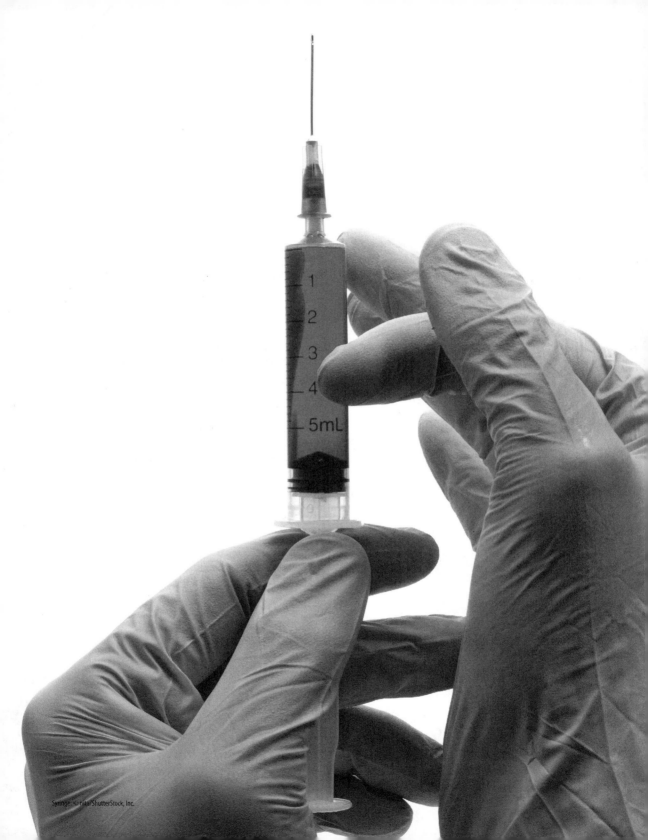

CHAPTER 4

IV Insertion

Melissa Kagarise, DHSc, PA-C, CLS

GOAL

► Demonstrate the knowledge and skills to successfully insert a peripheral intravenous (IV) catheter.

OBJECTIVES

1. Describe the indications and contraindications for IV placement.
2. Identify correct anatomic locations for IVs.
3. List supplies needed to perform an IV insertion.
4. Demonstrate correct technique for preparing and inserting an IV.
5. Recognize possible complications.
6. Discuss post-procedure follow-up related to IV placement.

RATIONALE

- Peripheral intravenous catheterization is a procedure utilized to gain direct access to the venous system in order to administer fluids, medications, and blood products, providing continuous access for therapy over an extended period of time.
- Administering therapy through this means avoids the need for absorption through the gastrointestinal system, allowing for 100% bioavailability directly through the circulation.[1]

EVIDENCE-BASED INDICATIONS

- Administration of fluids
- Rapid delivery of medications
- Administration of blood and blood products

CONTRAINDICATIONS

- Peripheral IV cannulation should not be initiated in an extremity where there is edema, burns, sclerosis, phlebitis, or thrombosis. Attempting to infiltrate therapy through these areas will substantially increase the risk of infection and **extravasation**, and can result in suboptimal volume flow.
- Areas with cellulitis, shunts, or fistulas should be avoided in order to decrease the risk of bacteremia or thrombosis.
- IVs should not be started on the ipsilateral side of a radical mastectomy or where there is significant trauma to the neck, chest, or abdomen where the venous return system may be compromised.[2]

COMPLICATIONS

- Complications of peripheral IV insertions can range from minor discomfort and localized hematoma formation to systemic infections. Local complications at the site of IV insertion include discomfort at the site, ecchymosis, and hematoma formation.

- **Infiltration** occurs when the IV catheter has become dislodged from the vein or when there has been a perforation of the vein that allows fluids to accumulate within the tissue. Signs of infiltration include a reduction in the infusion flow and edema at the site, with skin temperature that will feel cool to the touch.
- Phlebitis, acute inflammation of the vein, can occur with prolonged IV therapy. Early research documented increased incidence of phlebitis when IVs were inserted in the forearm using smaller catheter sizes and IV dwell times greater than 36 hours. This early research supported routine catheter changes every 24–36 hours.[3] Recent research has found that the incidence of phlebitis is not substantially different when comparing routine changes every 3 days to changing IV site when clinically indicated.[4,5] In 2011, the Centers for Disease Control and Prevention (CDC) published guidelines recommending rotating peripheral IV catheter sites no earlier than 72–96 hours. Catheter sites should be evaluated daily and require change only if there are clinical signs of **phlebitis** (warmth, tenderness, erythema, or palpable cord). The CDC continues to evaluate evidence to determine whether recommendations will support the move to changing IV sites only when clinically indicated.[6] Practitioners should follow their employment protocol for IV care.
- Local infection, bacteremia, and septicemia can result as a consequence of a break in **aseptic technique** during insertion or handling of sterile equipment. Pain, swelling, erythema, and purulent discharge may be noted. Catheter, air, and pulmonary emboli may occur due to incorrect IV insertion techniques.

SPECIAL CONSIDERATIONS

- Pediatric and geriatric populations deserve special consideration when considering IV therapy. In the pediatric population, venous access most commonly is attained through superficial veins in the dorsum of the hand. Additional sites for IV access include the antecubital fossa, dorsum of the foot, and—in newborns—the scalp.[2] IV cannulation should utilize the smallest catheter size to accommodate the vessel selection and therapy and may include the use of a butterfly catheter.

- Geriatric patient populations require special mention regarding IV therapy. Physiological changes as an individual ages make elderly patients more susceptible during invasive procedures and fluid therapy. Wall tone of the veins can be weaker and more tortuous, making the vessel more fragile and susceptible to rupture, or may be more sclerotic and distended, making insertion more difficult.[7] Changes in the skin and connective tissue make the vein more prone to rolling when trying to directly insert a catheter into the vein. Loss of subcutaneous tissue results in veins becoming prominent and tortuous; the use of tourniquet can increase venous congestion, resulting in increased blood leakage around the puncture site. Using a blood pressure cuff instead of a tourniquet can help to decrease this risk. Utilizing the smallest gauge of catheter, lowering the angle of approach, and adequately stabilizing the vein can help improve procedure success. In addition, when securing the IV to the skin, care must be taken not to disrupt fragile skin.

SUPPLIES

- Personal protective equipment: gloves
- Sharps container and trash receptacle
- Tourniquet or blood pressure cuff
- Antiseptic antimicrobial swabs/pads
  - Chlorhexidine gluconate
  - Povidone-iodine
- Sterile gauze
- Sterile, transparent, semipermeable dressings
- Adhesive tape
- IV pole, IV solution, and administrative set

FIGURE 4-1: Vascular access supplies

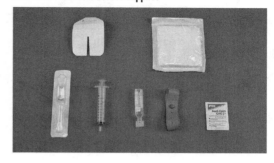

- 2 needles/cannula: butterfly or Angiocath (size dependent upon therapy)
  - 24 gauge and butterfly (pediatric population)
  - 20–22 gauge (typical IV fluid and medication administration)
  - 16–18 gauge (blood and blood product administration)
- Local anesthetic as needed
- See **FIGURE 4-1**

PROCEDURAL INSTRUCTIONS

- Verify the patient and procedure to be performed.
- All supplies should be collected and placed near the patient (see **FIGURE 4-2**).
- Prior to starting an IV, hands should be washed and gloves should be put on for protection.
- Selecting the appropriate vein for IV access includes consideration of the following

FIGURE 4-2: Prepare IV insertion supplies

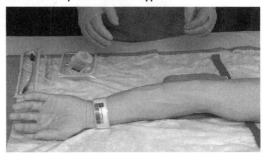

factors: location for best access, type of therapy, and rate of infusion. Always begin with the distal veins and work proximally; begin with the dorsal metacarpal veins of the hands or the cephalic, basilic, and median veins of the arms.

- The dorsal metacarpal and cephalic veins are most commonly used, because they provide good venous access, interfere least with patient mobility, and have a decreased risk of phlebitis as compared to vessels in the lower extremity.
- The patient should be positioned comfortably and in such a way that allows full access to intended placement site.
- Prepare and assemble the IV fluid and tubing by first verifying the intended medication, inspecting the solution for clarity, and noting expiration date.
- Patient consent for the procedure should be obtained and allergies should be verified.
- Remove administration set (tubing) from the packaging, inspect the integrity of the tubing, and ensure the clamp is in the closed position.
- Remove the protective cap from the administration port on the solution bag and remove the protective cap from the tubing spike.
- Maintaining aseptic technique, squeeze the drip chamber and spike the solution bag with the tubing spike (see **FIGURE 4-3**).

- Hang the solution bag on a pole above the level of the patient's heart and fill the drip chamber halfway.
- Maintaining the sterility of the end of the tubing, remove the end cap (do not discard or drop) and open the tubing to expel air.
- Close the clamp and replace the protective cap at the end of the tubing without breaking aseptic technique.
- Place tubing within easy reach so that it can be attached to the catheter hub immediately upon cannulating the vein.
- Apply the tourniquet 8–10 cm above the intended IV insertion point to locate the most suitable veins.
- Palpate veins for stability and firmness; look for veins that are straight without palpable valves.
- Cleanse the area with the topical antimicrobial solution and allow the area to dry.
- Just prior to inserting the catheter, inspect the unit, ensuring that the catheter slides easily on the needle and the bevel is visible at the tip.
- Using the nondominant hand, grasp the forearm or hand and position the thumb just below the insertion point.
- In order to stabilize the vein, gently apply downward or distal pressure with the thumb to make the skin taut over the vein.
- Insert the Angiocath with the bevel up at a 15° angle directly into the vein (see **FIGURE 4-4**). A slight "pop" will be felt when the needle

FIGURE 4-3: IV fluid

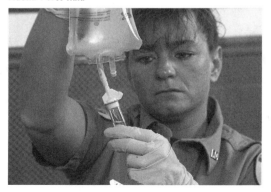

FIGURE 4-4: Apply tourniquet and insert IV catheter

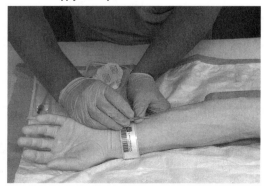

and catheter enter the vein; blood will flow into the flash chamber of the Angiocath.

- Lower the Angiocath angle to position the catheter hub close to the skin and advance 2–3 mm farther to ensure that the needle and catheter have both entered the lumen of the vein. With the nondominant hand, fully advance the catheter into the vein, keeping the needle held steady.

- Once the catheter has been advanced into the vein, release the tourniquet and apply light pressure to the skin just proximal to the catheter tip to prevent the leaking of blood back through the catheter.

- Remove the needle and dispose of it in the appropriate sharps container. Never try to reinsert the needle back into the catheter once it has been removed. This can cause a shearing of the catheter that may result in catheter emboli.

- Pick up the tubing with the dominant hand, pop off the protective cap, and attach the tubing to the catheter hub (see **FIGURE 4-5**).

- Once attached, the pressure over the proximal end of the catheter can be released to allow flow into the vein.

- While holding the catheter and tubing securely, open the tubing clamp and verify flow through the tubing and into the vein.

- Any blood within the flash chamber will clear as solution flows into the veins. Observe for signs of infiltration that could

FIGURE 4-5: Attach tubing to IV catheter

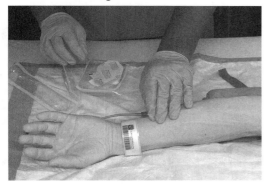

FIGURE 4-6: Secure IV tubing

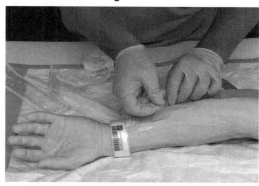

indicate improper venous catheterization, including reduction in the infusion flow, edema at the site, or skin temperature that is cool to the touch.

- Once proper placement and flow have been verified, the catheter can be secured. **Chevron taping** is commonly used to secure the catheter in place.

- A 4- to 5-inch length of ½-inch tape is placed adhesive side up under the base of the IV line and crossed over the hub to adhere to the skin on the opposite side.

- A 3-inch length of tape should be used to secure the distal end of the tubing to the skin (see **FIGURE 4-6**). Avoid placing tape directly over the insertion point of the catheter.

- Following institutional procedure, a transparent adhesive covering may be placed over the catheter insertion point, allowing for direct visualization of the skin.

- The tubing should be looped and secured to the skin in order to decrease tension on the catheter from patient movement (see **FIGURE 4-7**).

FOLLOW-UP CARE

- The IV site should be checked daily for signs/symptoms of infection including erythema, edema, and a burning or stinging sensation at the site. If noted, the IV should

FIGURE 4-7: Tape tubing in place

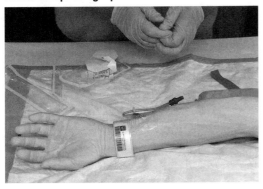

be removed and relocated. IVs should be changed every 72–96 hours[6] or as indicated by hospital protocol.

- When removing an IV, first clamp the tubing to stop the flow of solution into the vein. Remove the adhesive tape/dressings and lay sterile gauze over the insertion point of the catheter.
- Holding on to the hub of the catheter, swiftly pull the catheter out in one smooth motion.
- Apply pressure with sterile gauze at insertion point.

▶ REFERENCES

1. Ingram P, Lavery I. Peripheral intravenous therapy: key risks and implications for practice. *Nurs Stand*. 2005;19(46):55–64.

2. Liu SW, Zane R. Peripheral intravenous access. In: Roberts JR, Hedges JR, eds. *Roberts: Clinical procedures in emergency medicine*. 5th ed. Philadelphia: Elsevier Saunders; 2010.

3. Singh R, Bhandary S, Pun KD. Peripheral intravenous catheter related phlebitis and its contributing factors among adult population at KU teaching hospital. *Kathamandu Univ Med J (KUMJ)*. 2008;6(24):443–447. http://www.kumj.com.np/issue/24/443-447.pdf. Accessed October 5, 2012.

4. Rickard CM, Webster BA, Callis MC, et al. Routine versus clinically indicated replacement of peripheral intravenous catheters: a randomized controlled equivalence trial. *Lancet*. 2012;380(9847):1066–1074. Doi: 10.1016/S0140-6736(12)61082-4.

5. Rickard CM, McCann D, Munnings J, et al. Routine resite of peripheral intravenous devices every 3 days did not reduce complications compared with clinically indicated resite: a randomized controlled trial. *BMC Medicine*. 2010;8(53). http://www.biomedcentral.com/1741-7015/8/53. Accessed October 5, 2012.

6. O'Grady NP, Alexander M, Burns LA, et al. Guidelines for the prevention of intravascular catheter-related infections. *Clin Infectious Dis*. 2011;52(9):e162–e193. doi:10.1093/cid/cir257. http://www.cdc.gov/hicpac/pdf/guidelines/bsi-guidelines-2011.pdf. Accessed October 5, 2012.

7. Davis-Hall E. Inserting intravenous catheters. In: Dehn RW, Asprey DP, eds. *Essential Clinical Procedures*. 2nd ed. Philadelphia: Elsevier Saunders; 2007:71–82.

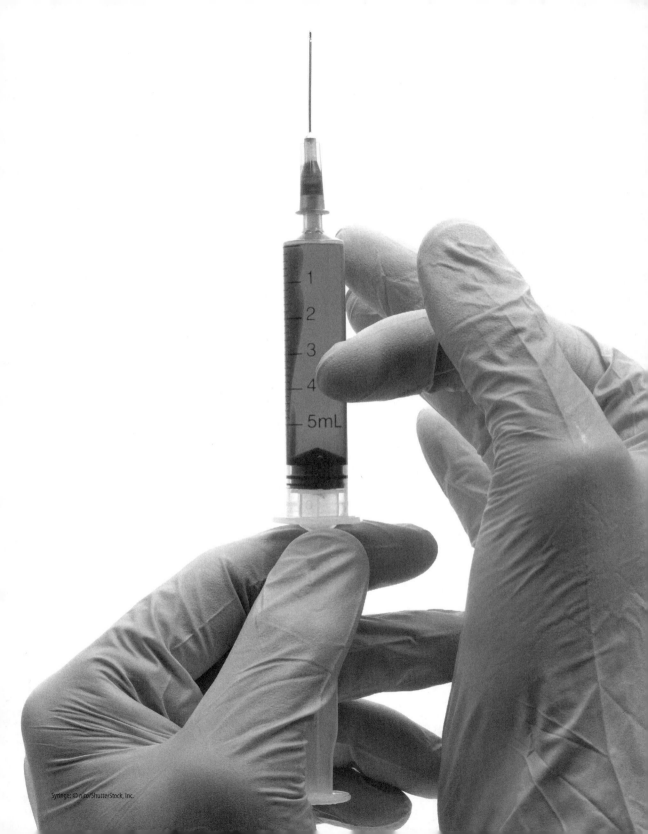

CHAPTER 5

Arterial Blood Gas

Jami S. Smith, MPA, MEd, PA-C

GOAL

▶ Obtain an arterial blood sample through arterial puncture with minimal injury to the patient.

OBJECTIVES

1. Identify the indications, contraindications, and complications of arterial puncture.
2. Describe how to perform an Allen test.
3. Identify the supplies needed for arterial puncture.
4. Describe the steps involved in obtaining an arterial blood sample via arterial puncture.

RATIONALE

- The sites for arterial puncture in adults are radial, brachial, and femoral arteries.
- The radial artery is preferred due to its superficial location and collateral circulation with the ulnar artery.
- Arterial puncture is a quick method of obtaining an arterial blood sample to assess the oxygenation and acid–base status of a patient.

EVIDENCE-BASED INDICATIONS

- To obtain information used to assess a patient's respiratory and metabolic acid–base status and the adequacy of oxygenation in the following conditions:
  - Respiratory distress
  - Management of ventilator-dependent patients
  - **Diabetic ketoacidosis**
  - **Metabolic acidosis** or **alkalosis**

CONTRAINDICATIONS

- Arterial puncture should not be performed if:
  - The radial pulse is non-palpable.
  - There is an overlying soft tissue infection.
  - The **Allen test** is negative, indicating there is no ulnar artery supply.
  - There is an arteriovenous fistula proximal to the intended site.
  - The patient has a severe coagulopathy.

COMPLICATIONS

- Arterial occlusion
- Bleeding
- Hematoma formation
- Injury to tendons and nerves

SPECIAL CONSIDERATIONS

- An Allen test should be performed to assess the collateral circulation before

FIGURE 5-1: Allen test

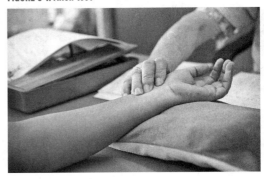

© Apples Eyes Studio/Shutterstock

performing the arterial puncture of the radial artery (see **FIGURE 5-1**). To perform the Allen test, elevate the extremity and apply pressure over both the distal radial and ulnar arteries at the level of the wrist on the volar surface. Release the pressure over the ulnar artery and observe for immediate flushing, which is indicative of a patent ulnar artery. This is considered a positive Allen test. If there is a negative Allen test (no flushing in the ulnar distribution), then repeat the test in the contralateral arm. If the test remains negative, then the arterial blood should be sampled from the femoral artery.[1]

SUPPLIES

- 3-mL **heparinized blood gas syringe** with capping device
- 21- to 25-gauge, $1/2$- to $5/8$-inch needle for arterial puncture
- Alcohol swab
- Sterile 2" × 2" gauze pad
- Label with patient name, date, time, and respiratory status
- Sterile gloves
- 1% lidocaine without epinephrine
- Syringe and 25- to 27-gauge needle for local anesthesia infiltration

FIGURE 5-2: Palpate radial artery

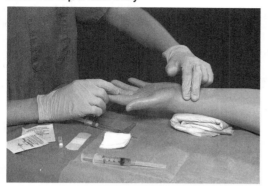

FIGURE 5-3: Inject area with lidocaine

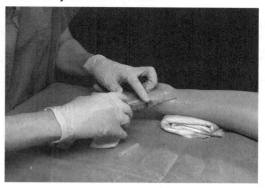

PROCEDURAL INSTRUCTIONS

- Explain the procedure to the patient and obtain verbal consent.
- The patient should be positioned in a comfortable position, either sitting or supine. The forearm should be supinated with a rolled towel under the forearm to gently elevate and extend the wrist. The Allen test should be performed to confirm patency of the ulnar artery prior to performing radial artery puncture.
- Palpate the radial artery just proximal to the wrist to determine the site of prominence of the radial artery (see **FIGURE 5-2**).
- Cleanse the overlying skin with alcohol.
- Anesthetize the overlying skin with 1% lidocaine.[2]
- Palpate the radial artery with the non-dominant index and long fingers to confirm site of maximal pulsation.
- Attach the 21- to 25-gauge needle to the heparinized syringe and hold the syringe in the dominant hand.
- Insert the needle into the anesthetized skin at the site of maximal impulse just until a blood flash is seen in the hub of the needle or lower portion of the syringe (see **FIGURE 5-3**). Once the needle has entered the radial artery, the pulsations should fill the syringe without further manual suction required (see **FIGURE 5-4**).

FIGURE 5-4: Arterial puncture performed

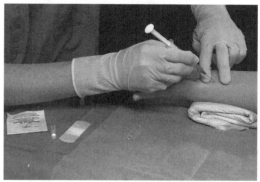

FIGURE 5-5: Remove air from syringe

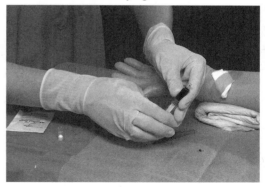

- Approximately 2–3 mL of blood should be collected; then, expel any air bubbles within the syringe (see **FIGURE 5-5**).[3]

- Remove the needle quickly in one motion, cap with device, and then apply a gauze pad with direct pressure to the affected area for at least 10 minutes and up to 20 minutes, depending on institutional guidelines.
- The blood should then be transported immediately to the laboratory with appropriate label attached. If not analyzed within 20 minutes, the specimen should be placed in wet ice for transportation.
- Recheck the site in 15 minutes to assess for adequate reperfusion of hand, hematoma formation, or continued bleeding.[2]

► REFERENCES

1. Pagana KD, Pagana TJ. *Mosby's Manual of Diagnostic and Laboratory Tests*. 5th ed. St. Louis: Elsevier Health Sciences; 2014.

2. Partin WR, Dorroh C. Emergency procedures. In: Stone CK, Humphries R, eds. *CURRENT Diagnosis and Treatment Emergency Medicine*. 7th ed. New York: McGraw-Hill Professional; 2011.

3. Milzman D, Janchar T. Arterial puncture and cannulation. In: Roberts JR, Hedges JR, eds. *Roberts and Hedges' Clinical Procedures in Emergency Medicine*. 6th ed. Philadelphia: Elsevier Saunders; 2014.

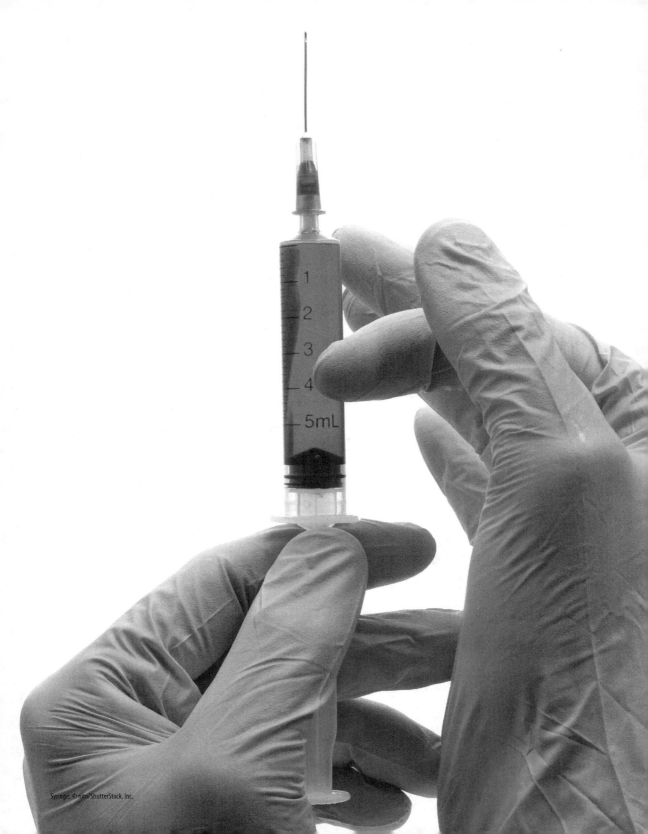

CHAPTER 6

Injections

Melissa Kagarise, DHSc, PA-C, CLS

GOAL

► Demonstrate the knowledge and skills to effectively administer intradermal, subcutaneous, and intramuscular injections.

OBJECTIVES

1. Describe the indications and contraindications for injections.
2. Identify the correct anatomic position for injections.
3. List supplies needed to perform injections.
4. Detail the appropriate needle length and gauge for each injection.
5. Demonstrate correct technique for administering intradermal, subcutaneous, and intramuscular injections.
6. Recognize possible complications.
7. Discuss post-procedure follow-up for intradermal injections.

RATIONALE

- Injections are utilized to administer a number of diagnostic and therapeutic medications. This form of parenteral administration includes intradermal, subcutaneous, and intramuscular routes of administration.

EVIDENCE-BASED INDICATIONS

- Diagnostic purposes in testing for hypersensitivity to allergens or infectious processes, including tuberculosis, via the intradermal route
- Therapeutic purposes, including insulin therapy via the subcutaneous route, and medication delivery via the intramuscular route when delivery of medication is needed with an intermediate rate of onset (10–30 minutes)[1]
- Disease prevention through vaccinations administered via the intramuscular route

CONTRAINDICATIONS

- Injections should not be administered on areas of skin with dermatitis, cellulitis, or scarring.
- An absolute contraindication for any injection is a documented allergy to the medication that is to be administered.

COMPLICATIONS

- Discomfort or pain at the injection site may occur. Allowing the alcohol to dry after cleansing the skin will help to minimize any burning that may occur as the needle punctures the skin. Inserting the needle with a quick thrust through the skin will also aid in decreasing the pain of the injection. In order to minimize injection pain during intramuscular injections, ensure the patient's muscle is relaxed and, if not contraindicated, massage the muscle after the injection.
- Anaphylactic reactions may occur with injection solutions. It is important to verify patient allergies prior to placing the injection. Treatment for anaphylactic reactions is supportive in nature, utilizing reversal agents when applicable. Infection or even abscess formation could develop at the injection site, particularly if aseptic technique is not followed when giving injections.
- Lipohypertrophy of the subcutaneous fat may be a result of repeated subcutaneous injections in the same area. Factors influencing development of lipohypertrophy include duration of diabetes, body mass index, and increased number of daily injections.[2] It is important to educate patients on rotating injection sites when frequent injections are necessary, as in the case of insulin therapy.

SPECIAL CONSIDERATIONS

- The majority of inactivated vaccines for infant immunizations are administered intramuscularly, most commonly in the vastus lateralis muscle on the leg.[3]

SUPPLIES

- Medication: supplied in ampules, vials, or prefilled syringes
- Syringe of appropriate size for volume of therapy
  - Intradermal: 1-mL or tuberculin syringe
  - Subcutaneous: 2- to 3-mL syringe
  - Intramuscular: 2- to 5-mL syringe
- Needle: size selection based on depth of insertion and type of fluid therapy
  - Intradermal: 26- to 27-gauge, $1/2$- to $5/8$-inch needle
  - Subcutaneous: 24- to 32-gauge, $3/8$- to $5/8$-inch needle
  - Intramuscular: for adults 18- to 22-gauge, 1- to 2-inch needle
- Alcohol wipes
- Personal protective equipment: gloves
- Sterile gauze pads
- Self-adhesive bandage
- Sharps container for needle disposal

PROCEDURAL INSTRUCTIONS

- All injection supplies should be collected and placed near the patient. Prior to performing an injection, hands should be washed and gloves should be applied for personal protection. Before administering an injection, the patient should be correctly identified and allergies should be documented. Verification of the appropriate medication and dose should be completed and patient consent obtained.
- Injection medications may be prefilled in the correct syringe or may require the practitioner to draw up the medication from an ampule or vial. Begin by assembling the appropriate needle and syringe for the injection. When withdrawing medication from an ampule, hold the ampule in the upright position, making sure all medication is at the bottom. The top of the ampule should be snapped off (glass) or twisted off (plastic). Insert the needle into the ampule, aspirate the medication, and then remove the needle and syringe.
- When drawing medication from a vial, air should be drawn into the syringe equaling the amount of medication that will be withdrawn. Cleanse the top of the vial with an alcohol pad, insert the needle into the vial top, and inject the air into the vial. Proceed with aspirating the required amount of medication into the syringe. Pull the needle from the vial and remove any air bubbles from the syringe.

Intramuscular Injections

- Intramuscular injection sites include the deltoid, gluteal, and vastus lateralis muscles. Due to the rich blood supply of the muscles, absorption of medications is fairly rapid, ranging from 10 to 30 minutes.[1] Muscle selection is dependent upon the age of the patient, solution type, and amount to be administered.
- Deltoid injections are typically utilized for patients age 3 years and older because of the ease of access and decreased risk for complications.[3] In order to avoid injury to the brachial artery and radial/ulnar nerves, the correct needle injection point within the deltoid muscle is located 2 to 3 fingerbreadths below the acromion process. The patient should be in a sitting position with the deltoid muscle relaxed and exposed.
- The gluteal muscle can be an injection site when there is a larger volume of solution required due to its larger size. Viscous material and volumes larger than 2.5 mL up to 5 mL should be given in the gluteal muscle. The injection site is located in the upper outer quadrant within the gluteus medius muscle in order to avoid injury to the sciatic nerve. Research suggests that injury to the sciatic nerve may be more common when using the dorsogluteal site as opposed to the ventrogluteal site for injection.[4] Positioning of the patient can be lying on the left or right side with area exposed. Location of the proper gluteal injection site begins by placing the palm of the hand over the greater trochanter, pointing the thumb toward the groin. With fingers pointed toward the patient's head, place the index finger on the anterosuperior iliac spine and the middle finger along the iliac crest, to form a "V" with the fingers. The injection point is located in the center of the "V."
- The vastus lateralis muscle is the preferred injection site for patients between the age of infancy and 2 years.[3] This large muscle is ideal, because it lacks major blood vessels and nerves. This muscle is located in the anterolateral thigh, one handbreadth below the greater trochanter of the femur to one handbreadth above the knee. Positioning of the patient can be sitting or lying with the muscle relaxed and exposed.

Once the site has been determined for an intramuscular injection:

- Prep the skin with a sterile alcohol pad using a concentric circular pattern (see **FIGURE 6-1**).
- Allow the alcohol to dry completely before proceeding in order to avoid introduction

FIGURE 6-1: Prep the skin using concentric circles

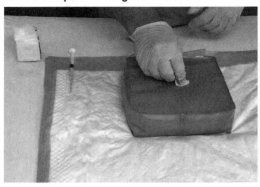

of the alcohol into the subcutaneous tissue and subsequent burning sensation with the injection.

- The skin should be held taut with the non-dominant hand to decrease the subcutaneous fat at the insertion point.
- The prepared needle and syringe should be quickly thrust through the skin into the muscle at a 90° angle or perpendicular to the skin (see **FIGURE 6-2**).
- Keeping the needle in the muscle, use the nondominant hand to pull back slightly on the plunger of the syringe and **aspirate** for blood (see **FIGURE 6-3**). If no blood is aspirated, slowly begin to inject the medication. If blood is aspirated, do not inject the medication and immediately withdraw needle and confirm correct position.

FIGURE 6-2: Insert needle at a 90° angle

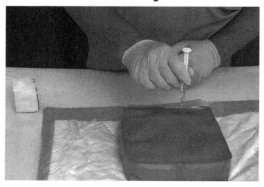

FIGURE 6-3: Pull back on plunger to check for blood with non-dominant hand

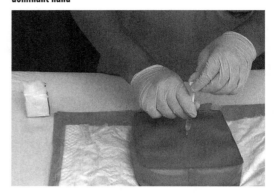

- Once all medication has been dispensed, quickly remove needle from skin, maintaining the 90° angle.
- Place a sterile gauze pad over injection site and lightly massage area to promote medication absorption, unless contraindicated with the type of medication dispensed (see **FIGURE 6-4**).
- Cover with a self-adhesive bandage.
- The needle/syringe should be disposed of in the appropriate sharps container system.

Intradermal Injections

- Intradermal injections are utilized in testing for hypersensitivity to allergens or infections (including tuberculosis). The injection is placed within the outer layers of

FIGURE 6-4: Place gauze or bandage on injection site

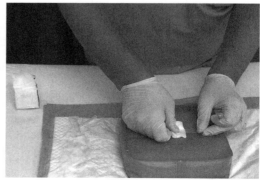

the skin where there is very little systemic absorption, allowing for observation of the local effects of the injected material. The site of injection is most commonly located in the ventral forearm, 3–4 finger widths below the antecubital space and 1 hand width above the wrist.[1] For extensive testing circumstances, the upper arms or back may be used.

- Position the patient in a sitting position with the extended forearm resting on a flat, firm surface.
- Prep the skin with a sterile alcohol pad using a concentric circular pattern.
- After the skin has dried completely, grasp the forearm and pull the skin taut with your thumb.
- With the bevel of the needle facing up, insert the needle at a 5° to 15° angle just into the dermis, approximately ⅛ inch. The needle tip should be visible below the skin surface.
- Slowly inject the antigen into the skin, forming a wheal.
- Remove the needle and dispose of it in the proper sharps container system.
- Do not rub injection site or place adhesive bandages over injection site. Observation of the local reaction to the injected antigen occurs over the next couple of days.

Subcutaneous Injections

- Subcutaneous injections deliver medication to the fatty tissue below the skin where absorption and delivery of medication occur in a slow but consistent manner. Insulin, anticoagulants, tetanus toxoid, allergy medications, and epinephrine are the most common formulations given via the subcutaneous route.[1] Insulin needle gauges are thinner and typically in the range of 28–32 gauge. The higher the needle gauge, the thinner the needle, resulting in less discomfort with the injection. Subcutaneous injection sites are located in areas where there are more subcutaneous fat stores: lower abdomen, triceps, anterior thigh, and scapular region.

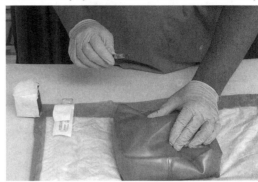

FIGURE 6-5: Grasp injection site and hold needle with the bevel up

- Position the patient in a comfortable position with injection site exposed.
- Prep the skin with a sterile alcohol pad using a concentric circular pattern.
- After allowing the alcohol to dry, the skin should be pinched with the nondominant hand (see **FIGURE 6-5**). This helps to pull the subcutaneous tissue up from the muscle, aiding in penetration into only the adipose tissue.
- With the bevel up, the needle of the prepared injection should be inserted at a 45° angle into the pinched skin and adipose tissue (see **FIGURE 6-6**).
- Advance the needle ¾ of the way into the skin.
- Keeping the needle within the skin and subcutaneous tissue, the nondominant hand

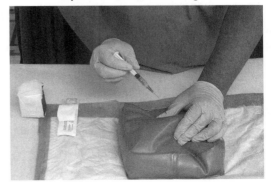

FIGURE 6-6: Prepare to insert needle at 45° angle

FIGURE 6-7: Release pinched skin following needle insertion

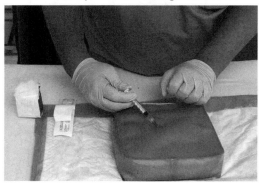

should release the pinched skin, allowing the tissue to relax (see **FIGURE 6-7**).

- Keeping the needle in the tissue, use the nondominant hand to pull back slightly on the plunger of the syringe and aspirate for blood. If no blood is aspirated, slowly begin to inject the medication. If blood is aspirated, do not inject the medication and immediately remove the needle.

- Remove the needle and syringe at the same angle of insertion and dispose of properly in a sharps container system.
- Cover the injection site with gauze and massage to facilitate absorption, unless contraindicated.

AFTERCARE INSTRUCTIONS

- A self-adhesive bandage may be placed over subcutaneous and intramuscular injections if there is minimal bleeding at the injection site. Due to the need for observation of the local reaction to the antigen from the intradermal injection, adhesive bandages or dressings should not be utilized.
- Patients should be told to contact the practitioner if they experience fever, pain, paresthesias, erythema, or discharge at the injection site.
- Patients receiving an intradermal injection should be instructed on the appropriate follow-up schedule with the practitioner for reaction evaluation, typically within 48–72 hours.

▶ REFERENCES

1. Gaylene A, Kerestzes P, Wcisel MA. Medication administration. In: Altman GB, ed. *Fundamental and Advanced Nursing Skills*. 3rd ed. Clifton Park, NY: Delmar Cengage Learning; 2010:593–613.
2. Omar MA, El-Kafoury AA, El-Araby RI. Lipohypertrophy in children and adolescents with type 1 diabetes and the associated factors. *BMC Res Notes*. 2011;4:290. doi:10.1186/1756-0500-4-290.
3. Centers for Disease Control and Prevention. *Epidemiology and Prevention of Vaccine Preventable Diseases. The Pink Book*. 13th ed. Public Health Foundation; 2012. http://www.cdc.gov/vaccines/pubs/pinkbook/downloads/vac-admin.pdf. Accessed October 4, 2012.
4. Small SP. Preventing sciatic nerve injury form intramuscular injections: literature review [abstract]. *J Adv Nurs*. 2004;47(3):287.

▶ ADDITIONAL READING

Centers for Disease Control and Prevention. Injection safety: CDC's role in safe injection practices. http://www.cdc.gov/injectionsafety/CDCsRole.html. Updated May 14, 2014. Accessed June 25, 2015.

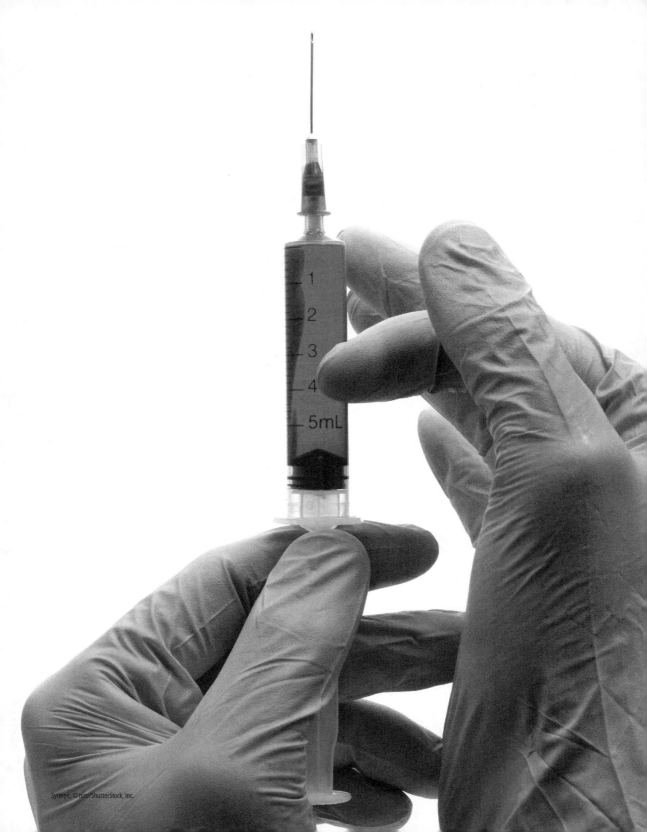

CHAPTER 7

Venipuncture

Adrian Banning, MMS, PA-C
Rosalie Coppola, MHS, PA-C

GOAL

▶ Obtain a **venous sample** of blood while observing universal precautions.[1]

OBJECTIVES

1. Describe the indications, contraindications, and rationale for performing **venipuncture**.
2. Identify and describe common complications associated with venipuncture.
3. Describe the essential anatomy and physiology associated with the performance of venipuncture.
4. Identify the necessary materials and their proper use for performing venipuncture.
5. Identify the important aspects of postprocedure care following venipuncture.

RATIONALE FOR PROCEDURE

- Blood can be collected from several veins, most commonly from the antecubital fossa of the anterior arm.[1–3]
- ✳ The most common site for drawing blood from the antecubital fossa is the median cubital vein; the basilic and cephalic veins are also used.[2,3] This vein is just medial of center in the antecubital fossa (see **FIGURE 7-1**). When looking at the anterior right arm, the median cubital vein is medial to the brachioradialis muscle and lateral to the medial epicondyl. It is a vein that joins the cephalic vein (lateral, anterior arm) and the basilic vein (which runs along the medial side of the anterior arm, medial to the biceps brachii body).[3–5]
- The median cubital vein lies superficially to the tendon and **aponeurosis** of the biceps brachii muscle, which is covered by antebrachial **fascia**.[4,5]
- Cubital lymph nodes are found proximally to the median cubital vein at the upper edge of the cubital fossa. Remember that venous blood returns to the heart from extremities in a distal to proximal flow.[4,5]

EVIDENCE-BASED INDICATIONS

- Laboratory diagnostic evaluation of blood to establish or exclude a diagnosis[3]
- Screening for a specific disease entity[2]

FIGURE 7-1: Right upper extremity venous system, antecubital fossa

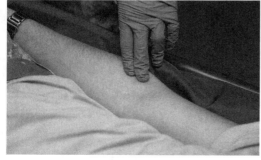

© Jones and Bartlett Publishers. Courtesy of MIEMSS.

- Determining therapeutic prognosis[2]
- Evaluating for complications of therapy[2]
- Determining therapeutic drug dosage and preventing drug toxicity[2]
- Blood transfusions[2]
- **Therapeutic phlebotomy** for the treatment of diseases including **polycythemia vera** and **hemochromatosis**[2]

CONTRAINDICATIONS

Contraindication limited only to site selection of the venipuncture:

- **Lymphedema**[2]
- Preexisting **thrombophlebitis**[2]
- **Dialysis shunt**[2]
- Skin infection[2]
- Severe vascular disease or venous obstruction[3]

COMPLICATIONS

- Infection[2]
- Bleeding[2]
- **Hematoma**[2]
- Fainting or dizziness[2]

SPECIAL CONSIDERATIONS

- Do not collect venipuncture samples from an arm where lymph node dissection has occurred. This could increase the risk of infection.[2,3]
- Do not collect blood from an arm that has an IV inserted. If necessary to do so, do not collect blood proximal to the IV insertion site.[1,2]
- Gently roll tubes or invert. Do not shake tubes too vigorously or for too long. This could damage the blood cells collected, causing hemolysis. No more than eight inversions of a tube are necessary.[2]

SUPPLIES

- Clean gloves
- Alcohol swab

FIGURE 7-2: Patient preparation

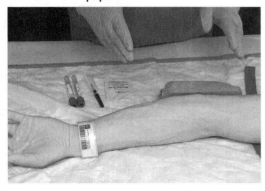

FIGURE 7-3: Blood collection supplies

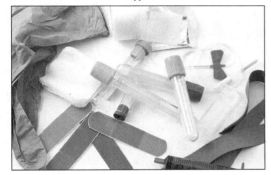

© PatCotilloJr/iStock

- Cotton swab
- Tourniquet
- Needle (18–21 gauge)
- Syringe (10–50 mL), if not using Vacutainer
- Adhesive bandage
- Collection tube(s): These tubes come topped with a variety of differently colored rubber stopper tops, indicating that they are used for different purposes or types of samples (plasma, chemistries, glucose, ammonia) and with different additives.[1–3]
- See **FIGURES 7-2** and **7-3**.

PROCEDURAL INSTRUCTIONS

- The patient should be identified and informed of the procedure and what types of samples are being collected.[2]
- Assemble all required equipment.[2,3]

- The patient should be advised that he or she may experience a pinching sensation when the needle used for collection enters the skin. Needles with larger numbers have smaller bores. Therefore, an 18-gauge needle has a larger opening than a 21-gauge needle. 21-gauge needles are commonly used in adult venipuncture.[3]
- The patient is placed in a comfortable seated position with the arm to be used for venipuncture raised and resting on a clean surface with the antecubital fossa exposed.[2,3]
- Request that the patient make a fist in order to make the veins of that arm more visible.[1–3]
- The person collecting the sample should wear new, clean gloves. Sterile gloves are not required.
- Apply a clean **tourniquet** several inches above the antecubital fossa.[1–3] Do not leave the tourniquet on for any more than 60 seconds. This could cause acid buildup in the sample.[2]
- Using a circular motion, starting from the inside and working outward, swab the skin with an alcohol solution to clean the skin where the venipuncture will occur (see **FIGURE 7-4**).[1,2]
- Allow the skin to dry for several seconds before inserting the needle.[1,2]
- Do not pat or blow on the area. Do not touch the skin after it has been cleaned.

FIGURE 7-4: Cleaning the skin

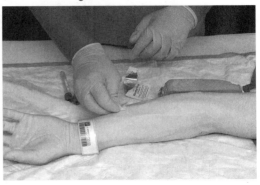

- Starting in the antecubital fossa, look and palpate for the vein to be used for blood collection. Palpate with the fingertip of the gloved, nondominant hand.[3] Veins appear blue under the skin.
- Provider will feel a resilient sensation in a vein; remember that veins do not have pulses. Venipuncture does not utilize arteries. Tendons will be cord-like.[3]
- Hold the needle, syringe, or Vacutainer in the dominant hand for insertion.[1,3]
- Insert the selected needle (needles vary in bevel size) with the bevel (opening) facing upward at approximately 15°–30° from the horizontal surface of the arm (see **FIGURE 7-5**). Stabilize the vein with the nondominant hand so that it does not move away from the needle or "roll." If inserted correctly, blood will flow into the Vacutainer once it is attached.[1-3]
- Once blood begins to flow into the Vacutainer or collection container or is withdrawn via syringe, remove the tourniquet.[1-4]
- If a vein in the antecubital fossa is not accessible or unsuccessful, you can try the veins on the dorsal surface of the hand. If the upper extremity is not an option, the femoral vein can also be used for blood collection.[1-3]

FIGURE 7-5: Needle insertion with bevel facing upwards

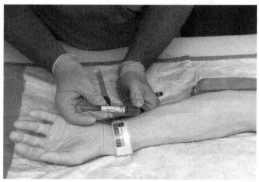

FIGURE 7-6: Remove the needle and apply gentle pressure

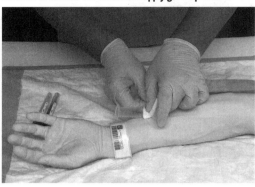

- Replace collection tube with another if collecting further samples.[3]
- When finished collecting samples, firmly place a cotton ball or gauze over the needle and carefully withdraw the needle, applying gentle pressure to the venipuncture site for 3–5 minutes (see **FIGURE 7-6**).[3] Bending the arm at the elbow is not necessary. Elevating the arm will also increase the speed of coagulation.[1]
- Dispose of the needle and any contaminated objects in an appropriate container, using universal precautions.[2]
- Properly label and store the samples.[2]
- Apply an adhesive bandage over the cotton ball to collect any slight leaking or oozing that may occur from the venipuncture site.[2] Overt bleeding should not be present.

AFTERCARE INSTRUCTIONS

- Gentle pressure at the site after the procedure for several minutes will minimize any hematomas (bruising) at the site, as will removing the tourniquet in an expedited manner.[1,2]

► REFERENCES

1. Gomella LG, Haist SA. Bedside procedures. In: Gomella LG, Haist SA, eds. *Clinician's Pocket Reference: The Scut Monkey.* 11th ed. New York: McGraw-Hill; 2007. http://accessmedicine.mhmedical.com/content.aspx?bookid=365&Sectionid=43074922. Accessed April 27, 2015.

2. Pagana KD, Pagana TJ. Blood studies. In: Pagana KD, Pagana TJ, eds. *Mosby's Manual of Diagnostic and Laboratory Tests.* St. Louis: Mosby/Elsevier; 1998.

3. Partin W, Dorroh C. Emergency procedures. In: Stone C, Humphries RL, eds. *CURRENT Diagnosis and Treatment Emergency Medicine.* 7th ed. New York: McGraw-Hill; 2011. http://accessmedicine.mhmedical.com/content.aspx?bookid=385&Sectionid=40357220. Accessed April 27, 2015.

4. Moore KL, Agur AMR, Dalley AF. Upper limb. In: Moore KL, Agur AMR, Dalley AF, eds. *Essential Clinical Anatomy.* 4th ed. Baltimore: Lippincott Williams & Wilkins; 2011.

5. Rohen JW, Yokochi C, Lutjen-Drecoll E. Upper limb. In: Rohen JW, Yokochi C, Lutjen-Drecoll E. *Color Atlas of Anatomy.* 5th ed. Philadelphia: Lippincott Williams & Wilkins; 2002.

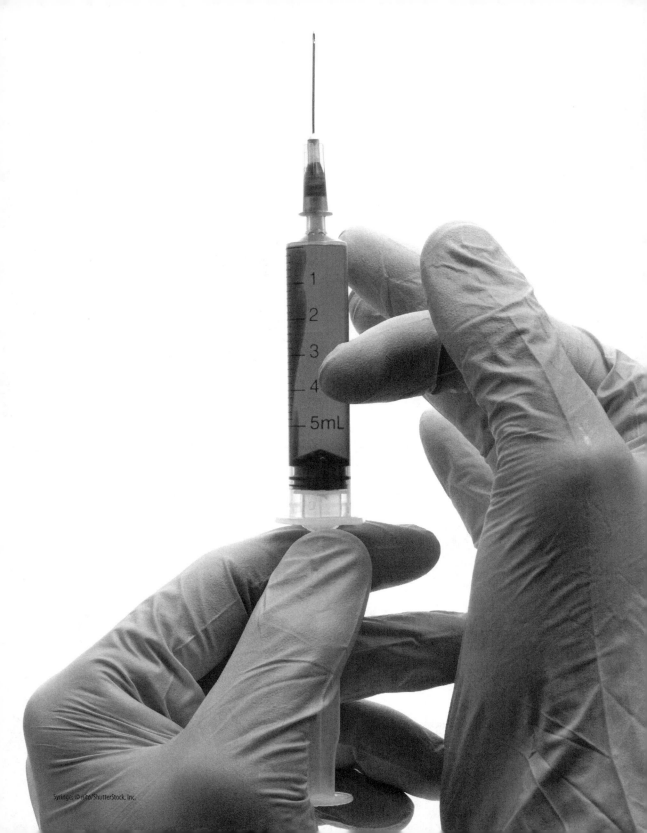

CHAPTER 8

Blood Cultures

Jami S. Smith, MPA, MEd, PA-C

GOAL

▶ Obtain high-quality venous blood sampling for the purpose of culture to detect bacteremia.

OBJECTIVES

1. Identify the indications, contraindications, and complications of blood culture collection.
2. Identify the supplies needed for blood culture collection.
3. Describe the steps involved in obtaining a venous blood sample for blood culture collection.
4. Understand methods for reducing contamination of blood culture samples.

RATIONALE FOR PROCEDURE

- **Bacteremia** can occur from thrombophlebitis, endocarditis, or hematogenous spread of bacteria from an infection from a distant source.
- Blood cultures are usually drawn in pairs to assist in the detection of contamination of the site.
- The blood is obtained via venipuncture at two different sites and transferred to two bottles, one for aerobic organisms (or **aerobic bacteria**) and the other for anaerobic organisms (or **anaerobic bacteria**). The bottles are incubated, and preliminary reports of growth can be detected at 24 hours. Final reports are usually available within 48–72 hours.

EVIDENCE-BASED INDICATIONS

- Blood cultures should be obtained prior to the initiation of antibiotic therapy in any patient suspected of bacteremia.
- Conditions for which blood cultures are especially important to their diagnosis and treatment include sepsis, meningitis, osteomyelitis, septic arthritis, endocarditis, pneumonia, and fever of unknown origin.[1]

CONTRAINDICATIONS

- There are no contraindications to obtaining blood cultures; however, contaminated cultures could result in the inappropriate use of antibiotics.

COMPLICATIONS

- Bleeding
- Hematoma formation
- Infection
- Injury to nerves, arteries, or veins

SPECIAL CONSIDERATIONS

- To avoid contamination, cultures should be obtained from venipuncture sites instead of **vascular devices**.[2]

- Multiple sets may be ordered and should be obtained from different sites.
- Blood cultures should be drawn prior to administering antibiotics; however, if the patient is already on antibiotics, then the blood cultures should be drawn shortly before the next dose is administered.[3]

SUPPLIES

- Tourniquet
- Gloves
- 70% isopropyl alcohol pads
- Povidone-iodine pads
- Laboratory request form and transport bags
- 2" × 2" gauze square
- 21-gauge needles and 20-mL syringe or vacuum tube adapter and needle
- Adhesive tape
- Aerobic and anaerobic blood culture bottles

PROCEDURAL INSTRUCTIONS

- Explain the procedure to the patient and obtain verbal consent.
- The patient should be positioned in a comfortable position either sitting or supine.
- Apply a tourniquet proximal to the collection site and palpate the vein from which the sample will be collected (see **FIGURE 8-1**).
- Cleanse the skin with alcohol and then again with povidone-odine pads in a circular, outward spreading motion and allow to

FIGURE 8-1: Place tourniquet and palpate vessel

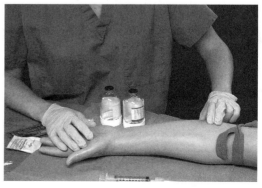

FIGURE 8-2: Cleanse site using circular motions

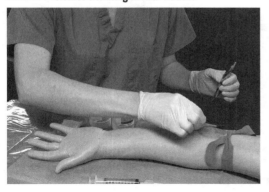

FIGURE 8-3: Perform venipuncture

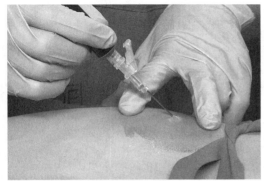

FIGURE 8-4: Apply pressure to site

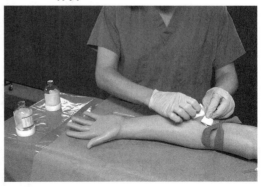

FIGURE 8-5: Place blood in bottle using sterile needle

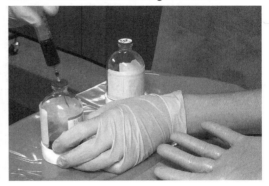

dry completely (see **FIGURE 8-2**). Also, cleanse the bottle tops with the povidone-iodine pads.

- Perform a venipuncture using a syringe or vacuum tube system (see **FIGURE 8-3**); draw 10 mL of blood.
- Remove the needle and tourniquet and then apply pressure to the site with gauze and adhesive tape (see **FIGURE 8-4**).

- Change the needle on the syringe and inject 5 mL of blood into each bottle (see **FIGURE 8-5**), then gently mix the contents.
- Label the specimens appropriately and send to the laboratory.

FOLLOW-UP CARE

No specialized instructions.

▶ REFERENCES

1. Reller LB, Sexton DJ. Blood cultures for the detection of bacteremia. *UpToDate.* April 17, 2015. http://www.uptodate.com/contents/blood-cultures-for-the-detection-of-bacteremia. Accessed July 9, 2015.

2. Kowalak J, ed. *Lippincott's Nursing Procedures.* 5th ed. Philadelphia, PA: Lippincott Williams & Wilkins; 2009:191–192.

3. Pagana K, Pagana T. Arterial blood gases. In: Pagana KD, Pagana TJ, eds. *Mosby's Manual of Diagnostic and Laboratory Tests.* 4th ed. St. Louis, MO: Elsevier; 2010: 114–124

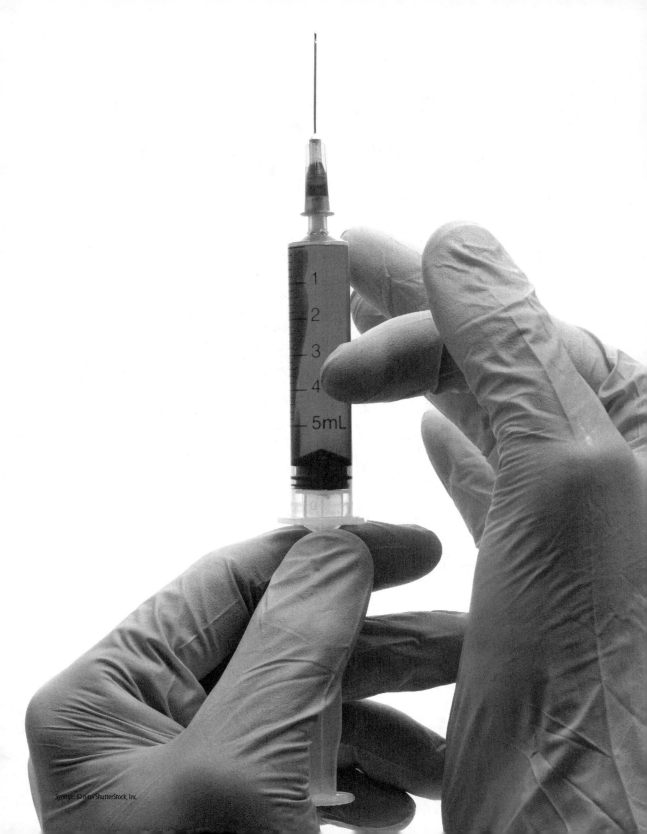

CHAPTER 9

Electrocardiogram Tracing

Deborah A. Opacic, EdD, MMS, PA-C

GOAL

▶ Perform an **electrocardiogram (ECG)** safely and accurately, and interpret the results of cardiac activity.

OBJECTIVES

1. Define the terms electrocardiogram, **monitor electrodes**, limb leads, and precordial leads.
2. Explain the clinical situations where an ECG would be indicated and provide rationales for each case.
3. Describe the contraindications to performing an ECG.
4. Identify and describe potential complications associated with performing an ECG.
5. Identify the materials necessary for performing an ECG.
6. Describe the steps for performing an ECG.

RATIONALE FOR PROCEDURE

- The ECG can identify the following pathology: evolving myocardial infarctions, myocardial ischemia, arrhythmias, various conduction defects, blocks, effects of hypertension on the heart muscle, effects of a pulmonary embolus on the heart muscle, electrolyte/metabolic derangements, pericardial inflammation, pericardial fluid, and cardiac effects from long-standing lung disease. The ability to successfully perform electrocardiography when clinically indicated is a necessary skill that all clinicians should acquire (see **FIGURE 9-1**).
- The ECG is a printed representation of the electrical activity of the heart created by recording the primary electrical event of contraction (depolarization) and the recovery phase (repolarization) of the myocardial tissue.
- **Positive depolarization** represents any electrical activity that moves toward the positive electrode. This results in a positive deflection above the isoelectric baseline. **Negative depolarization** represents any electrical activity that moves away from the positive electrode. This results in a negative deflection below the isoelectric baseline.
- The "12-lead" tracing is a three-dimensional view of the heart depicting all areas of the heart muscle. The 12 leads help to determine the location of **myocardial ischemia** or injury and the presence of chamber enlargement. A single-lead tracing helps to determine rhythm disturbances.

EVIDENCE-BASED INDICATIONS

- Subjective symptoms of:
  - Chest pain, palpitations, shortness of breath, nausea, diaphoresis, orthopnea, paroxysmal nocturnal dyspnea, dizziness, lightheadedness, syncope
- Objective findings of:
  - A new heart murmur, extra heart sound, irregular rhythm, heart rate too fast or too slow, pericardial rub, rales, edema, hypoxemia, hypotension, jugular venous distension, abnormal chest x-ray
- Baseline study in patients with high blood pressure, diabetes mellitus, chronic kidney disease
- Preoperative testing
- Electrolyte disturbances: potassium, calcium, magnesium
- Prior to exercise testing
- Ischemic heart disease
- Heart block
- Dysrhythmias
- **Myocardial hypertrophy**

CONTRAINDICATIONS

- Malfunctioning equipment
- Emergent need for airway, circulatory support
- Skin conditions that would interfere with lead placement

COMPLICATIONS

- Misinterpretation of the ECG
- Incorrect lead placement
- Skin irritation or damage from the electrode placement

FIGURE 9-1: ECG preparation

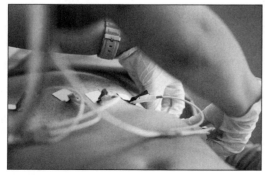

© ShotShare/iStock

SUPPLIES

- ECG machine
- ECG paper
- Electrodes
- Alcohol to clean skin surface

PROCEDURAL INSTRUCTIONS

Electrocardiogram Leads

- In preparation for performing a 12-lead ECG, an electrode is placed on each distal limb, and six leads are placed across the chest from right to left (see **FIGURE 9-2**).

Limb Leads (6)

- ECG machine automatically designates ± electrodes
- Frontal (coronal) plane view of the heart; view the electrical current moving up and down, left and right
- Three standard "bipolar leads"

Lead I	Right arm −	Left arm +	0°
Lead II	Right arm −	Left leg(s) +	60°
Lead III	Left arm −	Right leg(s) +	120°

FIGURE 9-2: Lead placement

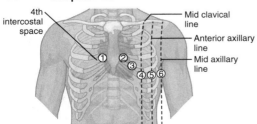

- Three augmented leads
  - Lead aVF is chosen to be positive, and leads aVR and aVL are negative.
  - The ECG machine amplifies (augments) the tracing for it to record

Lead aVL	Left arm +	Right arm −, Left leg −	−30°
Lead aVR	Right arm +	Left arm −, Left leg −	−150°
Lead aVF	Left leg +	Right arm −, Left arm −	+90°

- Representative views of the heart
  - Inferior   Lead II, lead III, lead aVF
  - Left lateral   Lead I, lead aVL
  - Right side (lateral)   Lead aVR

Precordial (Chest) Leads (6)

- Unipolar leads
- Anterior-posterior/horizontal view of the heart; view the electrical current moving anterior and posterior
- V_1–V_4 Anterior leads
- V_5–V_6 Left lateral leads

Steps

- Assemble the supplies, and make sure machine is operating correctly.
- Have patient remove jewelry (or anything metallic).
- Explain the procedure; instruct the patient to remain perfectly still during the tracing to avoid artifacts in the tracing.
- Wash hands.
- Verify patient and procedure.
- Position patient in supine position.
- Drape appropriately.
- Cleanse sites for lead placements.
- Attach limb leads identified on the individual machine lead placements.

- Attach **precordial leads** as follows:

Lead	Placement
V_1	Fourth intercostal space, just to the right of the sternum
V_2	Fourth intercostal space, just to the left of the sternum
V_3	Between V_2 and V_4
V_4	Fifth intercostal space, midclavicular line
V_5	Anterior axillary line, parallel with V_4
V_6	Midaxillary line, parallel with V_4 and V_5

- Standardize machine at 25 mm/sec (paper speed) by depressing the standardize button 1 mV/10 mm.
- Confirm all lead connections.
- Enter patient information.
- Ask patient to lie quietly.
- Press the record button auto for 12 lead, or choose the lead strip indicated.
- Review tracing for accuracy.
- Interpret tracing.
- Remove electrodes.
- Dispose of used supplies.
- Document date, time, and complications of procedure.

► **ADDITIONAL READING**

Goldberger AL, Goldberger ZD, Shvilkin A. *Clinical Electrocardiography: A Simplified Approach*. 8th ed. Philadelphia, PA: Elsevier Saunders; 2013.

Goldberger A. Electrocardiography. In: Longo DL, Fauci AS, Kasper DL, Hauser SL, Jameson JL, Loscalzo J, eds. *Harrison's Principles of Internal Medicine*. 18th ed. New York, NY: McGraw-Hill Medical; 2012:1831–1839.

Thaler MS. *The Only EKG Book You'll Ever Need*. 7th ed. Philadelphia, PA: Lippincott Williams & Wilkins; 2012.

White RD, Harris GD. Office electrocardiograms. In: Pfenninger J, Fowler G, eds. *Procedures for Primary Care*. 3rd ed. Philadelphia, PA: Elsevier Mosby; 2011:579–584.

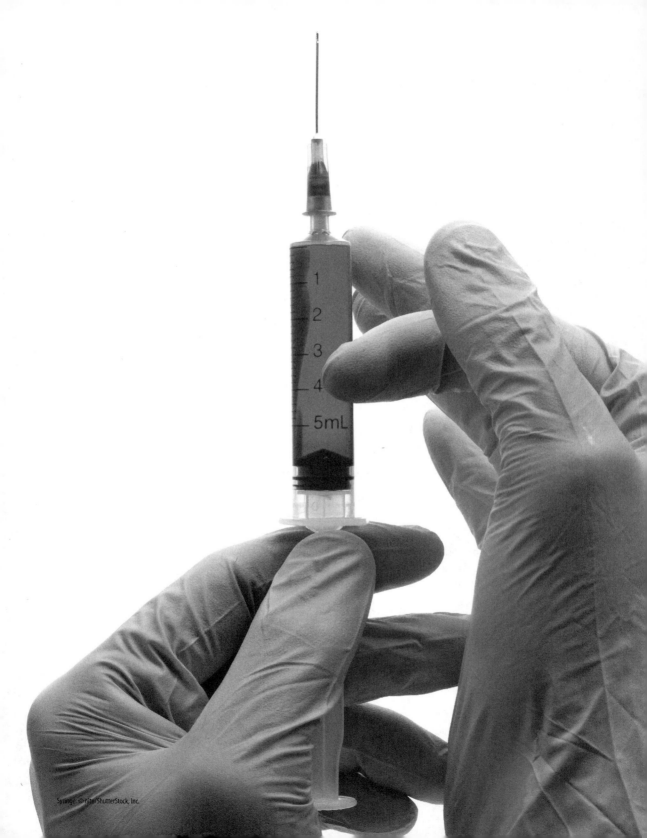

CHAPTER 10

Pulmonary Function Testing

Deborah A. Opacic, EdD, MMS, PA-C

GOALS

▶ Perform spirometry safely and accurately and interpret the results.

▶ Establish baseline lung function, evaluate dyspnea, detect pulmonary disease, monitor effects of therapies used to treat respiratory disease, evaluate respiratory impairment, evaluate operative risk, and perform surveillance for lung disease.

OBJECTIVES

1. Define pulmonary function tests and the following components used in pulmonary function testing:
   - Lung volumes: FVC, TLC, FRC
   - Measures of flow: FEV_1, $FEF_{25-75\%}$, **PEFR**, FEV_1/FVC, DLCO
2. Discuss the indications for spirometry.
3. Discuss the contraindications for spirometry.
4. Explain the procedure, including patient preparation.
5. List the equipment needed.
6. Describe the common complications of pulmonary function testing.

RATIONALE FOR PROCEDURE

- Pulmonary function tests (PFTs) refer to an array of studies or procedures that may be performed to assess the respiratory system.
- Spirometry is only one of several methods used to evaluate the status of the respiratory system. Spirometry is the most commonly used screening study to assess airflow (timed volume), lung volumes, lung capacities, and airway reactivity. These parameters are most commonly measured by determining the patient's **forced vital capacity (FVC)**.
- Key expiratory parameters are:
  - FVC
  - **Forced expiratory volume (FEV$_1$)** (see **FIGURE 10-1**)
  - The FVC, FEV$_1$, and the FEV$_1$/FVC ratio are necessary for routine clinical use. The FEV$_1$/FVC ratio is expressed as a percentage. A low ratio indicates airflow obstruction. Spirometry can also quantify the diffusion ability of the alveolar capillary membrane (**DLCO**). The forced expiratory flow (FEF$_{25-75\%}$) measures the airflow over the middle half (25–75%) of the forced vital capacity and is selective of small airways disease.

EVIDENCE-BASED INDICATIONS

- Symptoms:
  - Shortness of breath, wheezing, cough, chronic sputum production, chest pain, orthopnea
- Exam findings:
  - Diminished breath sounds, expiratory slowing, wheezing, chest deformity, hypoxemia, hypercapnia, polycythemia, abnormal chest x-ray findings
- Preoperative evaluation in patients with underlying lung disease
- Smokers 45 years or older
- Determining the severity of pulmonary insufficiency in patients with lung disease to aid in prognosis
- Patients with related risks:
  - Occupation, smoke exposure, drug toxicity
- Measure response to therapy
- Bronchoprovocation—inhalational challenge:
  - This test is performed to identify airway hyperreactivity. Agents used include methacholine and histamine. If there is a 20% reduction in the FEV$_1$, the test is considered positive for airway hyperreactivity.

CONTRAINDICATIONS

- When ordering PFTs, the clinician must use caution in:
  - Children under 5 years old
  - Patients in respiratory distress
  - Patients with unstable cardiovascular status
  - Patients who are unable to correctly perform the procedure

FIGURE 10-1: Forced expiratory volume

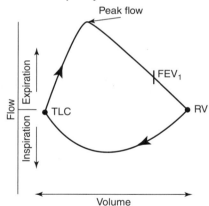

Flow-Volume Loop
- **Normal:** FVC, FEV$_1$, PEFR and FEF$_{25-75\%}$ >80% predicted; FEV$_1$/FVC > 95% predicted
  - Can be seen with intermittent disease (e.g. asthma), pulmonary emboli and pulmonary vascular disease
- **Obstructive:** Obstruction to airflow prolongs expiration
  - FEV$_1$/FVC <70% predicted and increased airway resistance and increased RV and TLC
  - Differential diagnosis: asthma, COPD, bronchiectasis, cystic fibrosis, bronchiolitis, proximal airway obstruction

Flow-Volume Loop
Restrictive: Reduced volumes without changes in airway resistance
- Decreased VC and TLC, FEV$_1$ and FVC decreased proportionately (FEV$_1$/FVC ratio >95% pred)
- Must confirm lung volumes by helium

- Unexplained hemoptysis
- Patients with cerebral, thoracic, abdominal aneurysms
- Patients who have undergone recent chest or abdominal surgery
- Patients recovering from recent eye surgery

SPECIAL CONSIDERATIONS

- Smokers should be instructed to abstain from smoking for at least 1 hour prior to testing.
- A clear explanation of the testing process is required for diagnostic accuracy.
- Watch the patient closely throughout the entire procedure, because he or she may become faint, lightheaded, dizzy, or short of breath.
- Factors known to influence the results of spirometry include:
  - Height
  - Age
  - Weight: truncal obesity restricts expansion of the chest cage; malnutrition causes reduced diaphragm strength, limiting the patient's ability to take a deep breath
  - Gender
  - Smoking history
  - Posture
  - Effort
  - Patient instruction

COMPLICATIONS

- Errors in measurement can be attributed to the following:
  - Inappropriate calibration of the machine
  - Air leak
  - Poorly fitted seal
  - Incomplete expiration
  - Poor initial expiratory effort
  - Patient not standing straight
  - Early termination
- The patient may become faint, lightheaded, dizzy, or short of breath.
- Poor effort may result in incorrect measurements.

FIGURE 10-2: Lung volumes

Lung volumes in a healthy individual

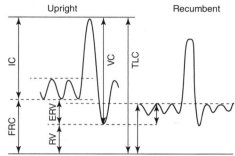

Abbreviations
ERV = expiratory reserve volume
$FEF_{25-75\%}$ = forced expiratory flow from 25–75% VC
FEV_1 = forced expiratory volume in 1 second
FRC = functional residual capacity
FVC = forced vital capacity
IC = inspiratory capacity
RV = residual volume
TLC = total lung capacity
VC = vital capacity
Spirometry Patterns
- Dilution or plethysmography (reduced FVC on spirometry not specific for restrictive disease, although normal FVC predicts normal TLC)
  - Differential diagnosis: interstitial disease, CHF, pleural disease, pneumonia, neuromuscular disease, chest wall abnormalities, obesity and lung resection
- **Bronchodilator response:** Positive if FVC or FEV_1 increase 12% and ≥200 mL
- **Poor effort:** Most reliably diagnosed by technician performing test rather than spirometric values. Forced expiratory time (FET) <6 seconds suggests inadequate expiration.

- Patients should perform no more than eight measurements in one sitting. Three measurements are the minimum.

Specific Measurements of Function

Lung Volumes (see FIGURE 10-2)

- Inspiratory reserve volume (IRV): Maximum amount of air that can be inspired in excess of the normal tidal volume
- Tidal volume (TV): Volume of air moved during a normal breath on quiet respiration
- Expiratory reserve volume (ERV): Maximum amount of air that can be exhaled in excess of the normal TV
- Residual volume (RV): Volume of air remaining in the lungs at the end of a maximal exhalation

Lung Capacities

- Inspiratory capacity (IC): The maximum amount of air a person can breathe in after a resting expiration
- Functional residual capacity (FRC): Volume of air in the lungs after a normal tidal expiration
- Vital capacity (VC): Maximum volume of air that can be exhaled from the lungs after a maximal inspiration
- Total lung capacity (TLC): Volume of air in the lungs after maximal inspiration; sum of all the volumes

EQUIPMENT NEEDED

- Spirometer
- Seating
- Nose clips
- Inhalants (bronchodilators)

PROCEDURAL INSTRUCTIONS

- There are two types of respiratory efforts: forceful (FVC) and relaxed (synchronized vital capacity [SVC]). SVC effort is not used routinely. SVC effort can be used in clinical situations where forced breathing is impossible. With this approach, the patient breathes normally, inhales fully, and then exhales fully to their ability; tidal volume is measured. The goal of the FVC effort is to measure the flow and volume of air.
- Assure that the spirometer is calibrated correctly. Machine calibration varies depending upon instrument used.
- Choose the spirometer settings; specific protocol (i.e., "PCP"—primary care practitioner protocol).
- Select adult or pediatric patient.
- Document patient position.
- Prepare the machine to test for FVC.
- Select FVC parameters: FVC, FEV_1, $FEV_{1\%}$, $FEF_{25-75\%}$ (depending on the indication for testing).
- Select effort type: FVC, FVU post*.
- Select curve: flow/volume; volume/time.
- Enter patient data into all mandatory fields:
    - Patient ID, name
    - Height

- Gender
- Race
- Age
- Smoke years
- Health history
- Medications
- Review/change the description of interpretations (mild, moderate, severe, very severe).
- Instruct the patient to:
    - Loosen any tight clothing, remove dentures.
    - Apply the nose clip (patient may pinch his or her nose).
    - Insert the mouthpiece, forming a tight seal with the lips.
    - Avoid bending forward when blowing.
    - Avoid blocking the transducer with the tongue.
    - Keep chin up.
    - Breathe in and out several times with nose clips in place to become familiar with the process.
    - Take as deep a breath as possible.
- Press start.
- Ask the patient to inhale fully, then exhale forcefully as fast and as long as he or she can (6 seconds) until FVC flattens out.
- When finished, have the patient breathe in as deeply as possible for inspiratory measurement.
- This may be repeated for a maximum of eight tries. Three tries is the minimum.
- The spirometer will stop automatically when breathing has stopped.
- Review data and accept or reject the interpretation. Review the interpretation and accept or reject the effort.
- Print test results.
- Determine reversibility of abnormal findings, administer bronchodilator, wait 15 minutes, and rerun the testing.
- Print test results.
- Dispose of used supplies.
- Document date, time, and complications of procedure.
- The results of the two largest FVC and FEV_1 values should be within 0.2 liter of each other to be considered acceptable.

▶ ADDITIONAL READING

Altman MA. Pulmonary function testing. In: Pfenninger J, Fowler G, eds. *Procedures for Primary Care*. 3rd ed. Philadelphia, PA: Elsevier Mosby; 2011:599–605.

Nagler J, Krauss B. Devices for assessing oxygenation and ventilation. In: Roberts JR, ed. *Robert and Hedges' Clinical Procedures in Emergency Medicine*. 5th ed. Philadelphia, PA: Elsevier Saunders; 2014:23–38.

Naureckas ET, Solway J. Disturbances of respiratory function. In: Longo DL, Fauci AS, Kasper DL, Hauser SL, Jameson JL, Loscalzo J, eds. *Harrison's Principles of Internal Medicine*. 18th ed. New York, NY: McGraw-Hill Medical; 2012:2087–2094.

Qaseem A, Wilt TJ, Weinberger SE, et al. Diagnosis and management of stable chronic obstructive pulmonary disease: a clinical practice guideline update from the American College of Physicians, American College of Chest Physicians, American Thoracic Society and European Respiratory Society. *Ann Intern Med*. 2011;155:179–191.

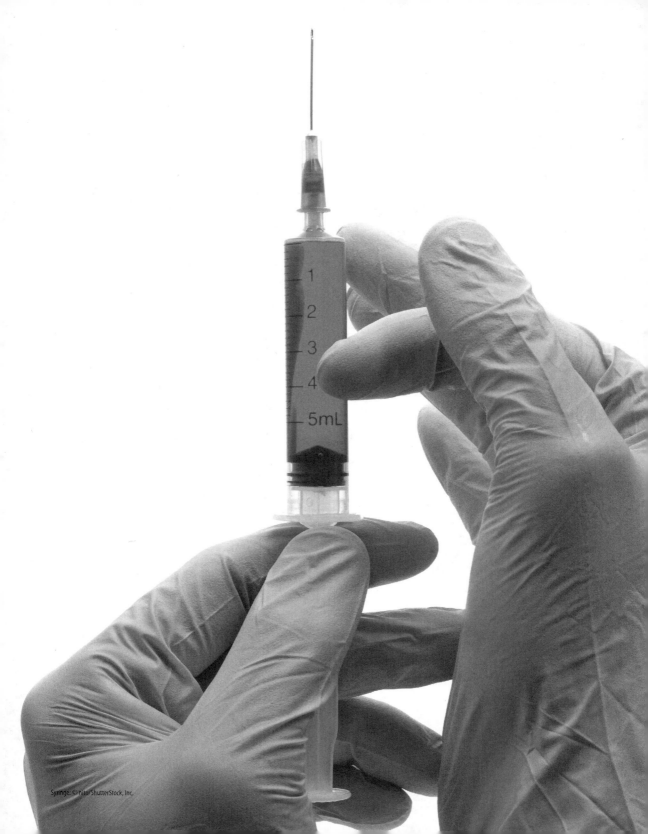

CHAPTER 11

Wound Closure and Management

Michelle L. Heinan, EdD, MS, PA-C
Patrick Auth, PhD, MS, PA-C

GOAL

► Decrease tissue loss, promote wound healing, and minimize scar formation.

OBJECTIVES

1. Describe the indications and contraindications for wound closure.
2. Describe the common complications associated with wound closure.
3. Describe the types of wound closure.
4. Identify materials necessary for performing wound closure.
5. Identify the components of post-procedure care after wound closure.

RATIONALE

- Wounds can be closed with a variety of different mechanisms. Depending on the type of wound, patient, and location, there are indications and contraindications to those closures. It is important that the clinician complete a thorough history and physical examination prior to making any decisions regarding closure. This evaluation may mean bringing in a specialist to evaluate and handle the wound closure due to severe underlying damage.
- Some of the general factors to consider with a laceration include risk of infection, delay of healing, possibility of a foreign body in the wound, cosmetic appearance, and evaluation of tetanus immunization status.[1,2] In order to minimize infection or scarring, a wound should be closed within 8 hours. "Some wounds can be closed up to 24 hours after injury if the anatomic location is highly vascular (e.g., face, neck, and scalp). And the cosmetic appearance is an important consideration."[1]

WOUND HEALING PATHOPHYSIOLOGY

- **Inflammatory phase**: This phase is the body's natural response to the injury and lasts from day 1 of the injury to day 5 post-injury. After initial wounding, the blood vessels in the wound bed contract and a clot is formed. This phase is characterized by *rubor* (redness), *tumor* (swelling), *dolor* (pain), and *calor* (heat). In wounds closed by primary intention, this phase lasts 4 days. In wounds closed by secondary or tertiary intention, this phase continues until epithelialization is complete.
- **Proliferative phase**: This phase is characterized by fibroblast proliferation stimulated by macrophage-released growth factors; increased rate of collagen synthesis by fibroblasts, granulation tissue, and neovascularization; and gain in tensile strength. This phase starts approximately 4 days after the wound occurs and may last 42 days post-injury.
- **Remodeling phase**: This phase starts approximately 6 weeks after the wound occurs and may last 1 year post-injury. This phase is characterized by an increase in tensile strengths; scar flattens and loses its red appearance.

EVIDENCE-BASED INDICATIONS[1,2]

Consider the following for specific wound closure technique:

- Location
- Shape
- Tension area
- Decreased blood flow to the area
- Depth: exposes the underlying subcutaneous tissue and possibly muscles and tendons
- Jagged edge
- Flap laceration

SPECIAL CONSIDERATIONS[2]

- Prolonged bleeding after applying direct pressure
- Embedded foreign body
- Tendon or nerve involvement
- Compromised vascular status
- Factors that affect wound healing
- Factors that influence increased infection
- Patient history of medical conditions and/or medications
- Anesthetic of antibiotic reactions in the past

CONTRAINDICATIONS

- Patients with bleeding disorders (referral to surgeon)
- Difficult to anesthetize (referral to surgeon)
- Contaminated wound closure after a couple of days if no infection noted

- Possibly wounds that involve muscles, nerves, and tendons (referral to a surgeon)
- Type of wound such as an avulsion injury

COMPLICATIONS[2]

Complications Associated with Wound Closure

- Infection
- **Keloid** formation or scarring
- Loss of structure
- Loss of function
- Lack of a good cosmetic appearance
- Wound dehiscence
- Tetanus
- Hematoma
- Complications due to delayed suture:
  - Increased tension on wound
  - Suture markings
  - No eversion of the wound edges
  - Scarring
  - Possible necrosis

SPECIAL CONSIDERATIONS

Primary Closure[1]

- Also called primary wound healing or primary closure, wounds that heal by first intention are characterized as having been closed by approximation of wound margins or by placement of a graft or flap, or that were created and closed in the operating room. Primary closure is the best choice for wounds that are in well-vascularized areas.
- Indications for this type of closure include recently sustained lacerations that can be closed within 12 hours generally and within 24 hours on face; wounds that are clean, tension free, and have viable tissue.
- Suture, staple, adhesive, or tape.

Secondary Closure[1]

- Also called secondary wound healing or spontaneous healing, wounds that heal by second intention are characterized as having been left open and allowed to close by epithelialization and contraction. Wounds that are contaminated or infected are commonly managed with this type of closure.

Tertiary Closure[1]

- Also called tertiary wound healing or delayed primary closure, wounds that heal by third intention are characterized as too heavily contaminated for primary closure but appear clean and well vascularized after 4–5 days of open observation.
- Indications for this type of closure include infected or unhealthy wounds with high bacterial content, wounds with a long time lapse since injury, and wounds with a severe crush component with significant tissue devitalization. Wound edges are approximated within 3–4 days post-injury, and tensile strength develops as in primary closure.

Adhesives Used for Wound Closure[2]

Advantages of Steri-Strips™

- Take less time to close wound
- No local anesthesia required
- Painless

Disadvantages of Steri-Strips™

- Difficult to keep laceration closed if tension is put on wound during physical activity
- Does not adhere well to skin that is moist or oily
- Scarring
- Infection

Advantages/Indications of Tissue Adhesives

- Take less time to close the wound
- No local anesthesia required
- Less painful than sutures
- Can provide an antimicrobial barrier and water resistance to some degree
- Can be used on extremities (except the hands), face, torso

Disadvantages/Contraindications of Tissue Adhesives

- Cannot be used over joints due to movement
- Long lacerations
- Hands
- Infection
- Mucocutaneous junctions or anywhere bodily fluids are present

TYPES OF WOUND[2]

- Abrasions: Superficial layer of tissue is removed.
- Avulsions: A section of tissue is torn off (partially or totally).
- Lacerations: Tissue is cut or torn; there are sharply demarcated borders.
- Puncture: small opening of indeterminate depth.

SUPPLIES FOR SUTURING[1]

- Gloves
- Gauze square
- Tissue scissors
- Scalpel: #11
- Irrigation syringe
- Saline
- Dressings
- Adhesive tape
- Anesthesia supplies: lidocaine, 10-mL syringe, 18-gauge and 25-gauge needles
- Needle drivers
- Tissue forceps (or skin hook)
- Scissors
- Sterile drapes
- Sterile gloves
- Suture materials:
  - Absorbable: Chromic catgut (natural monofilament), Vicryl (synthetic braided), PDS II (synthetic monofilament)
  - Nonabsorbable: silk (natural braided), Ethilon (synthetic monofilament)
  - Suture size: Ear or eyelid—6/0; face, eyebrow, nose, or lip—5/0 or 6/0; hands and limbs—3/0 or 4/0; scalp, torso (chest, back, abdomen)—3/0 or 4/0; foot or sole—3/0 or 4/0

PROCEDURAL INSTRUCTIONS

Suture Techniques[1]

- Deep layer approximation
  - Serves two purposes: closes potential spaces and minimizes tension on the wound margins; use absorbable sutures with a buried knot
- Simple interrupted
  - Used on the majority of wounds; each stitch is independent
  - To assure the best results in placing simple interrupted sutures:
    - Take equal volumes of subcutaneous tissue from both sides.
    - The needle should enter the skin edge at an angle of 90° or greater, and the angle of exit should ideally be the same as the angle of entrance (see **FIGURES 11-1, 11-2,** and **11-3**).
- Simple continuous
  - Rapid and easy to remove, provides effective hemostasis, distributes tension evenly along length; can also be locked with each stitch (see **FIGURE 11-4**)
- Horizontal mattress
  - Useful for single-layer closure of lacerations under tension (see **FIGURES 11-5** and **11-6**)
- Vertical mattress
  - Useful for everting skin edges

FIGURE 11-1: Simple interrupted suture wound closure

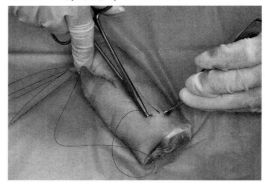

FIGURE 11-2: Simple interrupted suture

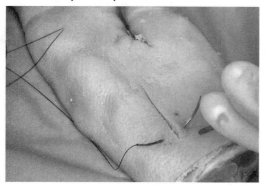

FIGURE 11-3: Completed simple interrupted suture

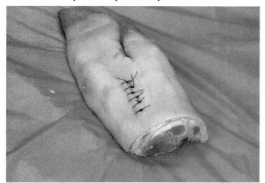

FIGURE 11-4: Continuous suture

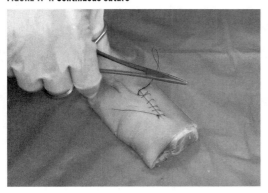

FIGURE 11-5: Suture placement for horizontal mattress suture

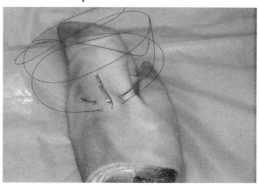

FIGURE 11-6: Completed horizontal mattress suture

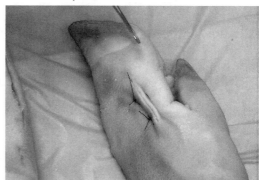

FIGURE 11-7: Needle placement

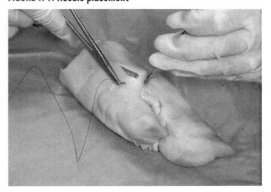

- Provides the best apposition and the best control of the wound edge (see **FIGURES 11-7** and **11-8**)
- The vertical mattress suture is basically a double suture that is made by passing

the needle more widely from the wound edges and deeper into the wound edges; this first suture loop will relieve the extrinsic tension from the wound edges and promote better healing (see **FIGURE 11-9**).

FIGURE 11-8: Vertical mattress suture

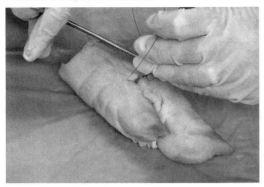

FIGURE 11-9: Completed vertical mattress suture

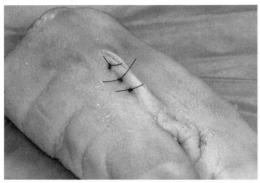

AFTERCARE INSTRUCTIONS

- See **FIGURE 11-10** for removal of simple interrupted stitches.
- Consult **TABLE 11-1** for average days before sutures can be removed for specific locations.
- Remove the bandage and gently wash around the wound every day.

FIGURE 11-10: Suture removal

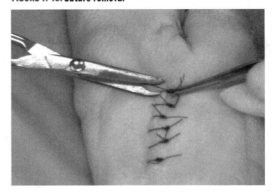

TABLE 11-1: Suture Removal Guide

Anatomic Location	Days (average)
Face	3–5
Arm (not joint)	7–10
Anterior trunk	10–14
Foot and hand	10–14
Joint	10–14
Scalp	10–14
Leg (not joint)	8–10

► REFERENCES

1. Newell K. Wound Closure. In: Dehn RW, Asprey DP, eds. *Essential Clinical Procedures.* 3rd ed. Philadelphia, PA: Elsevier Saunders; 2013:250–272.
2. Hollander JE, Singer AJ. Emergency wound management: evaluation of wounds. In: Tintinalli JE, Stapczynski JS, Cline DM, et al., eds. *Tintinalli's Emergency Medicine: A Comprehensive Study Guide.* 7th ed. New York, NY: McGraw-Hill Medical; 2011.

► ADDITIONAL READING

Dragu A, Unglaub F, Schwarz S, et al. Foreign body reaction after usage of tissue adhesives for skin closure: a case report and review of the literature. *Arch Orthop Trauma Surg.* 2009;129:167–16

Ediger MJ. Closure options for skin lacerations: evaluation and management. *Human Kinetics.* 2010;15(2):19–22.

Hoyt KS, Flarity K, Shea SS. Wound care and laceration repair for nurse practitioners in emergency care, Part II. *Adv Emerg Nurs J.* 2011;33(1):84–89.

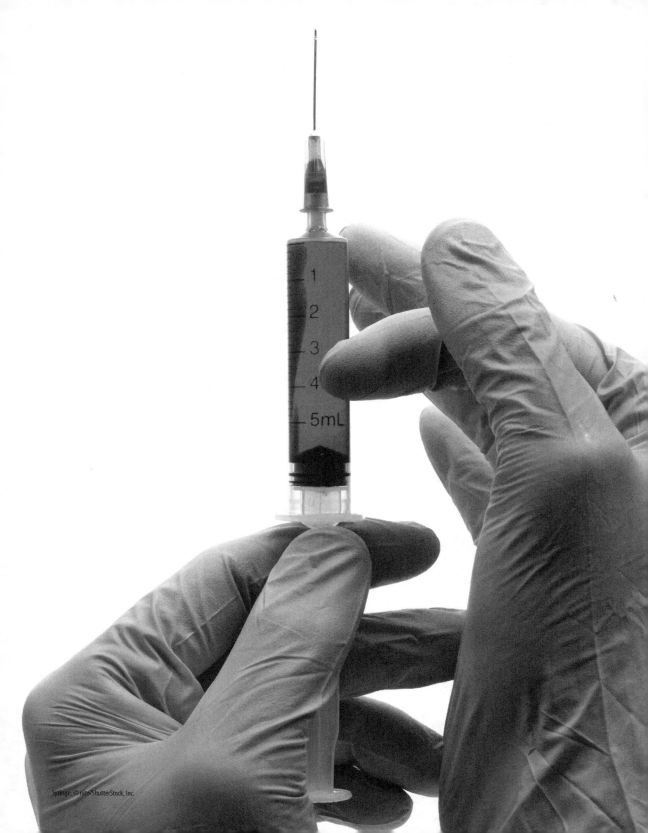

CHAPTER 12

Casting and Splinting

Daniela Livingston, MD, PA-C
Patrick Auth, PhD, MS, PA-C

GOALS

▶ Immobilize and protect orthopedic injuries.

▶ Prevent deformities.

OBJECTIVES

1. Describe the advantages and disadvantages of applying a splint and cast.
2. Distinguish the various types of splints and casts used to immobilize upper and lower extremity injuries.
3. Describe the indications for immobilization for upper and lower extremity splint and cast.
4. Identify and describe potential complications associated with casting and splinting of the extremities.
5. Describe how to apply a splint and cast.
6. Identify the important elements of patient education and cast care following a casting or splinting application.

RATIONALE[1]

- Casting and splinting serve to immobilize orthopedic injuries. They promote healing, maintain bone alignment, diminish pain, protect the injury, and help compensate for surrounding muscular weakness. Improper or prolonged application can increase the risk of complications from immobilization. Therefore, proper application technique and timely follow-up are essential.

EVIDENCE-BASED INDICATIONS

- The preferred initial treatment for fractures is realignment of the fractured bone(s) and splinting for immobilization. Other common methods of immobilization are casts and braces. The role of these methods is to maintain alignment, diminish pain, prevent further injury, and prevent muscular contractures.[1]
- Other than in cases of trauma, splints and casts may be indicated in congenital bone or joint deformities and neuromuscular abnormalities.[1]
- Splints are non-circumferential devices that can maintain the alignment of a limb with a fracture.[1] Splinting may be done in a variety of ways: folded sheets that can be used as **swathes** or slings, padded fiberglass, plaster slabs and pillows, or sandbags (for longer, stronger bones like the femur).
- One of the main roles of splinting is to prevent conversion of a **closed fracture** into an open one.
- Casts are closed and moldable devices that have a better fit on the immobilized limb (allow contouring over anatomic structures). Generally, limb casts have different shapes (transverse section): cylindrical for the forearm, square for the femur, and triangular for the leg.
- Before applying either a splint or a cast, patients have to be evaluated (in case of severe, multiple trauma) for airway, breathing, and circulation; the immobilized limb has to be examined for the quality of vascularization, innervations, and skin changes.
- Patient education is especially important in recognizing possible complications of immobilized, fractured limbs when using casts; it is essential that the patient moves fingers or toes to promote venous and lymphatic drainage.
- Conditions that benefit from immobilization include:

  - Fractures
  - **Sprains**
  - Severe soft-tissue injuries
  - Reduced **joint dislocations**
  - Inflammatory conditions: arthritis, **tendinopathy**, **tenosynovitis**
  - Deep laceration across joints
  - Tendon lacerations

CONTRAINDICATIONS

- Possible contraindications for casting are acute care of an **open fracture** or situations in which the patient cannot communicate if he or she experiences compression, abnormal pain, or numbness.

COMPLICATIONS[1]

- **Compartment syndrome**
- **Ischemia**
- Heat injury
- Pressure sores and skin breakdown
- Infection
- Dermatitis
- Joint stiffness
- Neurologic injury

ADVANTAGES OF SPLINTING

- Splints are faster and easy to apply.
- Splints prevent motion or help control motion of an extremity.
- Splints allow for swelling that occurs during the initial inflammatory phase of an injury.
- Preferred method of immobilization for acute injuries to prevent pressure-related

complications, such as pressure sores and compartment syndrome.

DISADVANTAGES OF SPLINTING

- Patient compliance
- Excessive motion at the injury site
- Splinting not suitable for fractures that are unstable or potentially unstable

ADVANTAGES OF CASTING

- Mainstay for treatment of most fractures
- Casts are a more effective method of immobilization

SUPPLIES[1,2]

- Adhesive tape (to prevent slippage of elastic wrap used with splints)
- Bandage scissors
- Basin of water at room temperature
  - Casting material hardens faster with the use of warm water compared with cold water. The faster the material sets, the greater the heat produced and the greater the risk of significant skin burns. Cool water is recommended when extra time is needed for splint application.
  - The dipping water should be kept clean and fresh. The temperature of the water should be tepid or slightly warm for plaster and cool or room temperature for fiberglass. These temperatures allow for workable setting time and have not been associated with increased risk of excessive heat production.
  - A good rule of thumb is that heat is inversely proportional to the setting time and directly proportional to the number of layers used.
- Casting glove is necessary for fiberglass
- Elastic bandage (for splints)
- Padding
- Stockinette
- Splinting and casting material is available in two types:

  - **Plaster of paris** (anhydrous calcium sulfate) is heavy and takes a long time to dry (24–48 hours).
  - **Synthetic plaster** (made of resin) is lighter and dries more quickly than plaster of paris (30 minutes to 1 hour).

PROCEDURAL INSTRUCTIONS[1]

General

- The healthcare provider should carefully inspect the involved extremity and document skin lesions, **soft-tissue injuries**, and neurovascular status before and after splint or cast application.
- Evaluate and document pulses, motor function, and sensory function to determine if emergency intervention or evaluation by a specialist is necessary.
- *Before* applying the splint or cast, drape the patient with a sheet or protective clothing.
- *Following* immobilization, neurovascular status should be rechecked and documented.

Basic Splinting Techniques

- Measure the amount of splint material needed. Lay the dry splinting material next to the injured body part to determine the length. The width of the splint should be slightly wider than the diameter of the body part being splinted.
- Soak the dry splinting material in a bucket of cool water. Wait for the splint material to stop bubbling.
- Take out the wet splint material and squeeze it gently. Excess water should be squeezed out and the plaster should still be wet.
- Smooth wrinkles out of the splint's layers, and make sure all the layers are flat.
- Put the wet splint material over the area being splinted; be sure to have the side of the splint material with the cotton padding closest to the patient's skin.
- Use one or more elastic bandages to secure the splint. The elastic bandages should

overlap approximately 25–50% with each layer.

- Mold the splinted part of the body into the desired position. Use the palms of your hands to mold the splint to the contours of the body part.
- Let the splint harden while holding it in the desired position.
- Finish the splint by applying adhesive tape along its sides. The tape will keep the elastic bandages in their place.
- Add a sling or provide crutches as necessary.

Basic Casting Techniques

- Apply a protective layer to the extremity with the use of a fabric stockinette (see **FIGURE 12-1**).
- The stockinette and casting widths are as follows: hands 2 inches wide, arms 2–4 inches wide, feet 3 inches wide, and legs 4–6 inches wide.
- Avoid wrinkles and cut a sufficient length to extend beyond each end of the cast. For an upper extremity cast, cut a small hole in the stockinette where it lies across the base of the thumb; the stockinette can be pulled over the digits.
- Place cotton padding material over the stockinette for comfort and to allow for swelling (see **FIGURE 12-2**). Wrap the cotton padding around the extremity, overlapping the previous layer of padding by 25–50% and placing two layers of padding (see **FIGURE 12-3**). The cotton material can be stretched or torn

FIGURE 12-1: Apply stockinette

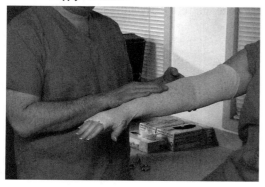

FIGURE 12-2: Application of cotton padding

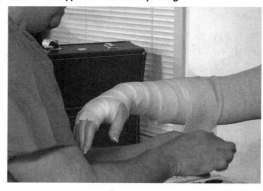

FIGURE 12-3: Application of padding around ankle

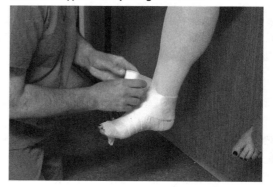

to allow uniform application. Avoid excessive padding or stretching, which can cause too much circumferential pressure.

- Pad the prominent areas smoothly and evenly without tension.
- Fill a bucket with lukewarm water and immerse the plaster material until it is saturated. Warm water will lead to faster drying of the plaster while cool water provides additional time for molding. Exothermic reaction will cause heat to be released as the plaster dries; thermal injuries may be prevented by avoiding water that is warmer than 50°C.
- Place the plaster over the padding (see **FIGURE 12-4**). Wrap the plaster. Roll evenly without tension, covering about one-third of the previous turn. Constant smoothing and molding are necessary to make the cast one whole and not a succession of layers (use palms) (**FIGURE 12-5**).

FIGURE 12-4: Application of casting material over padding

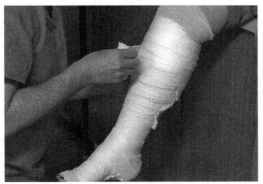

FIGURE 12-5: Fold stockinette over casting material

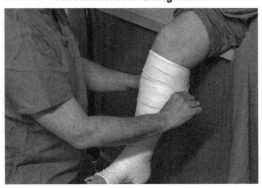

- Before the plaster dries, place the extremity in the desired anatomic position. Use the palm of your hands to mold the plaster gently to the extremity, taking care to avoid creating indentations that might lead to pressure points. Allow the cast to dry. Once the cast has dried, check for immobilization, anatomic positioning, strength of the cast, and patient comfort. Radiographs may be needed for fractures or dislocations that required reduction before cast placement.
- The plaster must be observed regularly for cracking, softening, or breakdown.

TABLES 12-1 through 12-4 identify the most commonly used splints and casts and their applications.

AFTERCARE INSTRUCTIONS

- Reevaluate the extremity immediately after completing the splint or cast application.
- Evaluate and document distal motor and sensory function, pulses, and color of the distal extremity, and assess capillary refill.
- Routine care after the application of a splint or cast should include extremity elevation,

TABLE 12-1: Most Commonly Used Splints[2]

Splint	Indications
Radial gutter	Fractures of the 2nd and 3rd metacarpal, flexor tendon or extensor tendon repairs
Ulnar gutter	Ulnar collateral ligament strain, triangular cartilage injuries, 4th and 5th metacarpal fractures
Volar (see FIGURE 12-6)	Wrist sprain, carpal tunnel syndrome, lacerations, triquetral fracture or lunate dislocation, 2nd through 5th metacarpal head fractures
Thumb-spica (see FIGURE 12-7)	Navicular/scaphoid and lunate fractures, thumb dislocations, proximal thumb fractures, ulnar collateral ligament sprains, de Quervain tenosynovitis
Sugar tong	Fractures of the distal radius, wrist, and forearm
Long-arm posterior	Stable fractures of forearm, fractures of elbow, sprains and dislocations of the elbow
Posterior lower leg (see FIGURE 12-8)	Distal tibial/fibular fracture, ankle sprain, ankle fractures, Achilles tendon tears, metatarsal fractures

FIGURE 12-6: Volar sprint

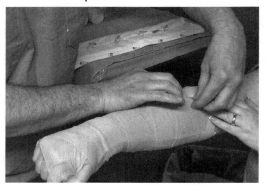

FIGURE 12-8: Lower leg splint

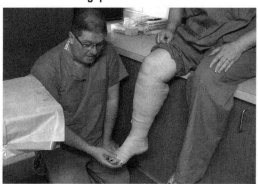

FIGURE 12-7: Thumb-spica splint

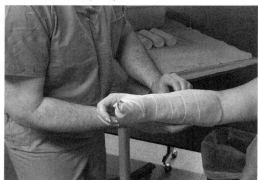

administration of medications for pain, and appropriate instructions for medical follow-up.

• Instruct the patient to keep the splint or cast clean and dry. As a general rule, it is recommended that any circumferential cast be checked the day after application for signs of circulatory compromise. If the cast is too tight, one must remember to split the plaster and the cotton padding.

• The patient should be informed to return for further evaluation if there are signs of neurovascular compromise or a compartment syndrome, such as swelling, worsening pain, discoloration of the distal extremity, difficulty moving fingers or toes, or a change in sensory function.

• Observe the extremity for pallor, paresthesia, paralysis, persistent or increasing pain, and weakening or pulselessness.

TABLE 12-2: Most Commonly Used Casts

Cast	Indications
Thumb-spica	Navicular/scaphoid fractures, trapezial fracture, 1st metacarpal fracture, carpometacarpal arthritis, de Quervain tenosynovitis, ulnar collateral ligament sprains
Short arm	Simple fractures of the forearm, particularly incomplete fractures in children, stable distal forearm fractures, and metacarpal fractures
Below the knee	Fractures of the distal tibia and fibula, fractures of the talus; calcaneus, cuboid, navicular, cuneiform, and metatarsal bones of the foot; fractures of the foot; ankle dislocations

TABLE 12-3: Key Points in the Application of the Specific Splint

Splint	Key Points
Radial gutter	Application should be from tip of 3rd finger to 2 inches from the antecubital fossa (3 fingers); cut 2.5-inch hole for the thumb and tape edges; flex the metacarpals 45° (70–90° if distal) and wrist 20–30° extension.
Ulnar gutter	Application should be from the tip of the 5th finger to 2 inches from antecubital (3 fingers); be sure to pad between the 4th and 5th fingers, mold to position: metacarpophalangeal at 50–80° flexion to maintain positioning in distal, proximal, and distal interphalangeal joints in slight flexion, wrist at 20° of flexion.
Volar wrist (see FIGURE 12-9)	Application of the splint should be from the palmar crease to 2 inches (3 fingers) from the antecubital; 1-inch fold at the angle of the palmar crease, place the forearm in a neutral position with the thumb upward and the wrist at 20° of extension
Thumb-spica (see FIGURE 12-10)	Application of this splint extends from the tip of the thumb to the proximal forearm. Place the forearm in a neutral position with the wrist at 20° of extension and the thumb slightly flexed.
Long arm	Application of the splint prevents flexion and extension of the elbow and limits supination and pronation. It extends along the posterior area from the wrist to the proximal humerus. Place the elbow at 90° of flexion while maintaining a neutral position for the forearm and wrist.
Sugar tong	Application of this splint will immobilize the wrist and forearm and prevent supination and pronation of the forearm. The splint extends from the metacarpophalangeal joints on the dorsum of the hand, along the forearm, around the elbow, and back to the volar aspect of the mid-palmar crease. Place the elbow at 90° of flexion while maintaining a neutral position for the forearm and wrist.
Posterior lower leg	Place the splint 2 inches below the popliteal to 2 inches beyond the toes; fold 1 inch under toes, wrap from the distal to proximal (toes up), and use a figure 8 with tape to hold in position. Be sure to maintain the ankle at 90° and to keep the fibular head free in order to avoid compression of the peroneal nerve. Lower extremity splints are not designed to bear weight and the patient should use crutches.

FIGURE 12-9: Application of volar wrist splint

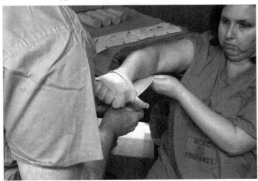

FIGURE 12-10: Application of thumb-spica splint

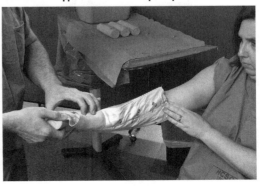

TABLE 12-4: Key Points in the Application of the Specific Cast

Cast	Key Points
Thumb-spica	The cast should allow for full elbow movement and should extend 2 inches from the antecubital to tip of the thumb.
Short arm	The cast should allow for full elbow movement and should not extend beyond the distal palmar crease to preserve motion of the metacarpophalangeal joints. The thumb should also maintain full range of motion and the wrist should be in a neutral position.
Below the knee	The ankle should be immobilized at a 90° angle, and the cast should not impede the range of motion at the knee.

► REFERENCES

1. Boyd AS, Benjamin HJ, Aspuld C. Principles of casting and splinting. *Am Fam Physician.* 2009;79(1):16–22.
2. Fitch MT, Nicks AB, Pariyadath M, et al. Basic splinting. *New Engl J Med.* 2008;359:32.

► ADDITIONAL READING

Coleman R, Reiland A. Orthopedic emergencies. In: Stone C, Humphries RL, eds. *CURRENT Diagnosis and Treatment: Emergency Medicine.* 7th ed. New York, NY: McGraw-Hill; 2011.

DeMaio M, McHale K, Lenhart M, et al. Plaster: our orthopaedic heritage: AAOS exhibit selection. *J Bone Joint Surg Am.* 2012;94(20):e152.

Iserson KV. Orthopedics. In: Iserson KV, ed. *Improvised Medicine: Providing Care in Extreme Environments.* New York, NY: McGraw-Hill; 2012:435–466.

Levy J, Song D, Judd D, et al. Outcomes of long-arm casting versus double-sugar-tong splinting of acute pediatric distal forearm fractures. *J of Ped Ortho.* 2013;28(6):1512–1520.

Philbin TM, Gittins ME. Hybrid casts: a comparison of different casting materials. *J Am Osteo Assoc.* 1999;99(6):311–312.

Simon RB, Brenner BE. *Emergency Procedures and Techniques.* Philadelphia, PA: Lippincott Williams & Wilkins; 1994.

Srinivasan RC, Tolhurst S, Vanderhave KL. Orthopedic surgery. In Doherty GM, ed. *CURRENT Diagnosis and Treatment: Surgery.* 13th ed. New York, NY: McGraw-Hill; 2012:435–466.

Williams KG, Smith G, Luhmann SJ, et al. A randomized controlled trial of cast versus splint for distal radial buckle fracture: an evaluation of satisfaction, convenience, and preference. *Ped Em Care.* 2013;29(5): 555–559.

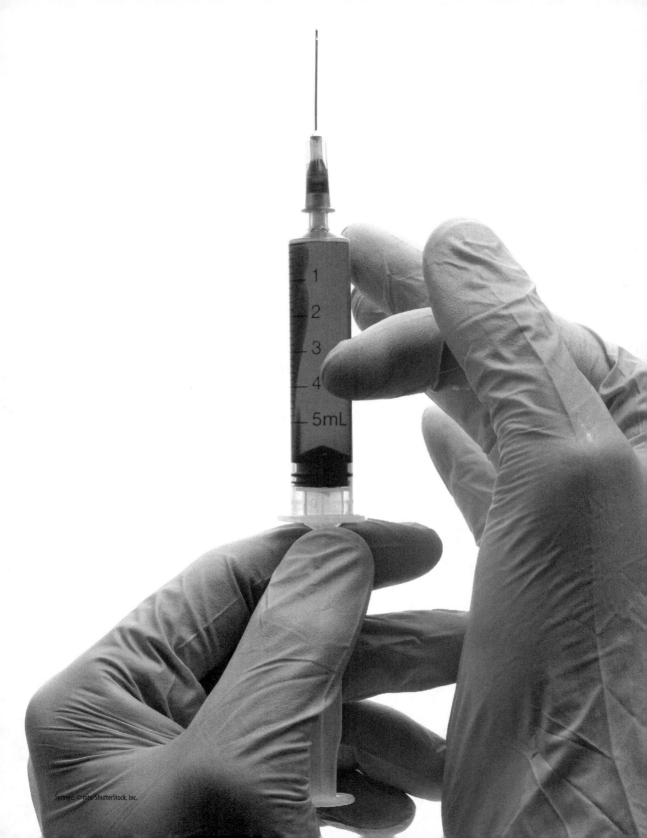

CHAPTER 13

Local Anesthesia

Joseph DiChiara, DO
Michael Green, DO

GOALS

- Induce local **analgesia** by injecting a drug into a specific part of the body.
- Prevent patients from pain sensation during medical procedures.

OBJECTIVES

1. Understand and explain the rationale for using local anesthetics, along with the benefits this modality provides for simple procedures.
2. Appreciate indications for local anesthetic use based on evidence-based scholarly activity.
3. Adequately evaluate and recognize various contraindications to the use of local anesthetics.
4. Identify complications associated with local anesthetic administration, along with the proper method of treating these complications.
5. Understand how the process of local anesthetic management differs in special populations and disease states.
6. Become familiar with the preparation, setup, supplies, and procedural steps required to safely and effectively administer local anesthetics.

RATIONALE FOR PROCEDURE

- The potential benefits and advantageous properties of local anesthetics have been recognized since the late 1800s, when cocaine, the first local anesthetic, was isolated and used for topical **anesthesia**. Since that time, numerous **ester** and **amide** local anesthetics have been developed for use in clinical practice.[1]
- The desire to develop local anesthetic compounds stemmed from the ability for these agents to produce a reversible loss of sensation when injected into a specific area of the body, thereby preventing or relieving painful stimuli. This is accomplished by the binding of these agents to voltage-gated sodium channels, ultimately resulting in the inhibition of nerve conduction in unmyelinated C fibers and small **myelinated** A fibers, both of which are responsible for transmission of pain.[2]
- Although numerous modalities are available for the prevention and treatment of painful stimuli, local anesthetics provide several distinct advantages. These include safe, simple, effective, and economical pain relief while avoiding the frequent side effects observed with narcotics, general anesthetics, and so forth. The implications for use of these compounds are vast; the compounds have been used successfully for many painful procedures such as skin surgery/biopsy, wound repair, abscess drainage, foreign body removal, lumbar puncture, and insertion of catheters. The ease of use combined with a wide application spectrum make local anesthesia an invaluable method for pain relief.[3]

EVIDENCE-BASED INDICATIONS

- Since their advent, local anesthetics have been used effectively in countless procedures, ranging from simple skin closure to the primary anesthetic used for surgical operations.
- The use of local anesthetics imparts the advantages of pain control during the procedure and short-term, postoperative pain relief while limiting the exposure and commonly encountered side effects of general anesthetics and narcotics. Although these agents cannot be used as the sole anesthetic for all procedures, they can be used in conjunction with the majority of pain control modalities used for most procedures.[3]
- Local anesthetics have been evaluated in multiple studies and compared against each other, along with other methods of pain relief. These studies have assessed their use for primary skin closure, superficial skin surgeries, orthopedic procedures, obstetric operations, abdominal surgery, hernia repair, facial surgery, and other procedures. Results show that, although not effective for long-term pain control, the benefits of pre-procedural pain relief, reduced intra-operative analgesic requirements, and short-term reduction of analgesics postoperatively make these compounds indicated for the majority of major and minor surgical procedures, either as the sole anesthetic or as adjunctive therapy to other methods of pain relief.[4-9]

CONTRAINDICATIONS

- Because adjuvant medications such as epinephrine are frequently coadministered with local anesthetics, contraindications to each injected medication must be identified.
- Local anesthetics are categorized into two groups, esters and amides, based on their chemical structure. Ester local anesthetics are metabolized by plasma cholinesterase, whereas amide local anesthetics are metabolized by hepatic microsomes. Therefore, atypical **pseudocholinesterase** and significant hepatic dysfunction are relative contraindications to the administration of esters and amides, respectively.
- Because most agents are renally excreted, renal dysfunction is a relative contraindication to local anesthetic use.
- An allergic reaction to one chemical classification of local anesthetic is a contraindication to the administration of another agent

in the same class; however, cross-reactivity between classes is minimal such that an agent in the other chemical class can usually be used safely.[10]

- Prilocaine has been associated with the development of **methemoglobinemia** and should therefore be avoided in patients diagnosed with this condition.[10]

- Patients being treated regularly with histamine antagonists have a reduced liver blood flow and should receive reduced dosages of amide anesthetics.[10]

- Anxiolytic medications should also result in reduced local anesthetic dosing, because these depressant medications can increase the depressive effects of local anesthetics.[10]

- Epinephrine is frequently coadministered with local anesthetics in order to produce vasoconstriction at the site of injection. Vasoconstriction causes a reduction in local blood flow, which reduces systemic absorption of local anesthetics. The result is prolonged local anesthetic duration of action, reduced likelihood of local anesthetic toxicity, and reduced blood loss at the site of injection. However, epinephrine has distinct contraindications related to conditions in which vasoconstriction would be unfavorable. These include uncontrolled high blood pressure, angina, coronary artery disease, diabetes, uncontrolled hyperthyroidism, pheochromocytoma, glaucoma, cocaine use within 24 hours, patients on nonselective beta blockers, and patients taking tricyclic antidepressants or monoamine oxidase inhibitors. In addition, epinephrine can lead to major ischemic complications if administered in the nose, ears, digits, or penis, especially in the presence of peripheral artery disease.[10]

COMPLICATIONS

- Over the years, local anesthetics have proven to be compounds that are exceptionally safe for administration, and their routine use has been employed for a large number of procedures. However, significant detriment has been linked to their utilization. Adverse reactions associated with these agents can be divided into systemic (toxic), localized, and allergic.[11]

- Systemic toxicity occurs when the blood level of a specific local anesthetic reaches a certain threshold. This threshold differs for each local anesthetic, meaning the maximum amount that can be safely administered is different for each compound. Systemic toxicity results in deleterious effects on the **central nervous system** (CNS) and cardiovascular system.

- Among the local anesthetics commonly used, bupivacaine has been shown to possess the greatest potential for systemic toxicity, especially for the cardiovascular system. Blood levels can reach this toxic threshold in multiple ways, including an unusually large dose, intravascular injection, slow biotransformation, or slow elimination. Methods that can be helpful in avoiding this potentially catastrophic occurrence include carefully aspirating prior to local anesthetic injection to decrease chances of intravascular injection, injecting slowly to recognize early signs of toxicity and abort further injection, and using the minimum amount of local anesthetic solution required to achieve adequate operative conditions.[11]

  - The first system to be affected by local anesthetic toxicity is the CNS. The severity of symptoms ranges from mild to severe depending on many different patient factors. Mild CNS toxicity presents as metallic taste, tinnitus, perioral numbness/tingling, sedation, slurred speech, mild tremors, disorientation, and visual/auditory disturbances. Moderate CNS toxicity presents as tonic-clonic seizures. Severe CNS toxicity includes coma, shock, and respiratory arrest. Treatment of CNS symptoms is supportive, with emphasis on airway control and symptomatic treatment until blood levels return to nontoxic levels.[11]

- At higher blood levels, local anesthetic toxicity results in negative effects to the cardiovascular system, resulting in significant myocardial depression and/or collapse. Cardiovascular side effects include bradycardia, atrioventricular block, arrhythmias, decreased myocardial contractility, and cardiac arrest. Treatment of cardiac symptoms involves employment of the advanced cardiac life support (ACLS) protocol, with intravenous lipid emulsion utilized for refractory conditions.[11]
- Localized reactions involve direct injury to connective tissue, neuronal tissue, or blood vessels at the site of injection, which results in pain, burning, paresthesias, hematoma, infection, edema, or paralysis. Chemical components of the injectate, needle trauma, or fast injection rates have been linked to these reactions. Proposed mechanisms to limit these reactions include preventing the number of needle penetrations, aspirating prior to injection, injecting slowly, and avoiding over-insertion of the needle.[11]
- Another complication involved in local anesthetic administration is the development of an allergic reaction. Although true allergies to local anesthetics are rare, there are reports of local anesthetic allergies, and a careful patient history is required to determine any such reaction. Esters are hydrolyzed into para-amino benzoic acid (PABA), which is the molecule responsible for the majority of allergic reactions. Therefore, because amides are metabolized by the liver and do not have PABA as a by-product, there are fewer allergic reactions with amides and they are more frequently used for local anesthesia. Skin testing by an allergist can be performed in order to determine if a true allergy exists prior to elective surgery; if there is a documented allergy and there is no time for allergy testing, a compound of the opposite class can be used because cross-reactivity does not commonly exist between chemical classes of local anesthetics.[11]

SUPPLIES

The healthcare provider should assemble the items needed for local anesthetic infiltration (see **FIGURE 13-1**). These include, but are not limited to, the following:

- Povidone-iodine or chlorhexidine solution
- Normal saline
- Sterile gauze
- Sterile gloves
- 25-, 27-, or 30-gauge hypodermic needle
- Syringe (1, 3, 5, or 10 mL)
- Local anesthetic agent (lidocaine, bupivacaine, ropivacaine)

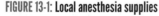

FIGURE 13-1: Local anesthesia supplies

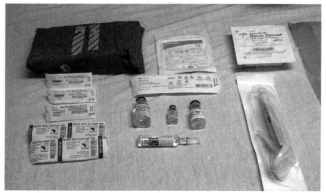

PROCEDURAL INSTRUCTIONS

- After the healthcare provider gathers all the pertinent patient information as previously discussed, the process of administering local anesthesia can commence.
- A discussion with the patient should occur, explaining the planned procedure and approach to be utilized; consent for the procedure must be obtained prior to the infiltration of any local anesthetic solution.
- An assessment of the area to be injected should be performed, taking into account the location, size/shape of wound, signs of infection, or preexisting neurovascular compromise.
- Using sterile gloves, the site is cleansed with povidone-iodine or chlorhexidine solution and allowed to air dry for the manufacturer's recommended duration of time (see **FIGURE 13-2**). Areas that are heavily contaminated prior to injection should be cleansed with normal saline solution prior to the application of sterile solution (see **FIGURE 13-3**).
- The anesthetic agent should be drawn up away from the patient in order to reduce any unnecessarily provoked anxiety.
- For intact skin, the needle is placed through the skin into the subcutaneous layer. For open wounds, the needle is placed into the subcutaneous layer by inserting it through the wound margin rather than through the intact skin.[3]
- Small volumes of local anesthetic are then injected slowly, advancing the needle forward and then withdrawing the needle throughout the injection (see **FIGURE 13-4**).

FIGURE 13-2: Don sterile gloves

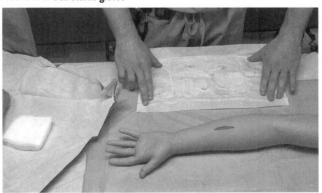

FIGURE 13-3: Prepare sterile field

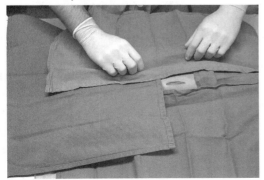

FIGURE 13-4: Inject anesthetic solution

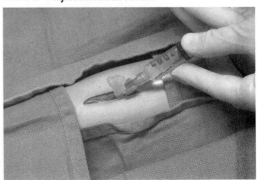

- Aspiration is usually not required, because the advancement and withdrawal of the needle reduces any significant amount of time the local anesthetic could be administered intravascularly.
- If adjacent areas require anesthetic placement, the needle is again inserted into previously injected skin in the direction of interest, and additional anesthetic is infiltrated. This serves to limit the amount of pain experienced from repeat needle insertions.
- Once the entire area of interest has been injected, the local anesthetic solution is given a few minutes to take action. The skin or wound margins are then tested for adequate anesthesia using a sharp object such as the needle used for local infiltration. If specific areas retain significant sensation, additional local anesthetic can be infiltrated into these specific locations.
- Once adequate anesthesia has been obtained, the patient is prepared to undergo the planned procedure.[3]

SPECIAL CONSIDERATIONS

- The injection of local anesthetics, although seemingly a benign and routine practice, must be performed in a careful and vigilant manner, taking into account the patient's medical history and comorbidities. In particular, a history of hepatic dysfunction, renal impairment, presence of atypical pseudocholinesterase, and disease states in which vasoconstriction would lead to increased risk of adverse outcomes should be sought and treatment adjusted based on these factors. Additionally, obtaining a basic understanding of the pharmacokinetics of local anesthetics—in particular the onset of action, duration of action, and maximum allowable volume to be injected—is prudent for safely and effectively administrating local anesthesia.
- Lidocaine has an onset of action between 2 and 5 minutes, with duration of action ranging from 30 minutes to 3 hours depending on whether epinephrine is coadministered. In comparison, bupivacaine has a slower onset of action, between 5 and 10 minutes, with duration of action up to 6 hours. The administration of epinephrine does not prolong the effects of bupivacaine owing to the intrinsic vasoconstrictive properties observed with bupivacaine administration. In addition, the mechanism of action of bupivacaine at myocardial receptor sites imparts an increased likelihood of cardiovascular depression and systemic toxicity. This information illustrates that various compounds can and should be used for specific purposes, and that one compound should not be used universally in all cases to achieve a specific outcome.[3]
- Administration of local anesthetics in children presents a specific challenge to the healthcare provider. As with any procedure in this population, anxiety regarding the process can severely limit the ability to effectively perform the task. Topical anesthetic techniques using EMLA (eutectic mixture of local anesthetics) cream or LET (lidocaine, epinephrine, tetracaine) can be very useful in calming the patient and his or her family, and can effectively reduce the initial pain on injection, which would otherwise minimize the ability to perform the local technique. If topical anesthesia is ineffective, procedural sedation may be required to effectively perform the procedure.[3]
- Local anesthetics have been used safely in pregnant patients and in patients who are breastfeeding. Caution is advised as to the use of epinephrine in this subset of patients, because concern for vasoconstriction and the effective blood supply to the fetus could theoretically be compromised. As with all other patients, using the lowest effective concentration of local anesthetics in this subset of patients can help avoid any deleterious side effects.[3]

► REFERENCES

1. Morgan GE, Mikhail MS, Murray MJ. Local anesthetics. In: Morgan GE, Mikhail MS, Murray MJ, eds. *Clinical Anesthesiology*. 4th ed. New York: Lange Medical Books; 2006.

2. Drasner K. Local anesthetics. In: Miller RD, Pardo MC, Jr, eds. *Basics of Anesthesia*. 6th ed. Philadelphia, PA: Elsevier Saunders; 2007.

3. Hsu DC. *Infiltration of Local Anesthetics*. http://www.uptodate.com/contents/infiltration-of-local-anesthetics. Updated February 17, 2015. Accessed July 9, 2015.

4. Ducarme G, Sillou S, Wernet A, et al. Single-shot ropivacaine wound infiltration during cesarean section for postoperative pain relief. *Gynecol Obstet Fertil*. 2012;40(1):10–13. doi: 10.1016/j.gyobfe.2011.07.035

5. Demiraran Y, Albayrak M, Yorulmaz IS, et al. Tramadol and levobupivacaine wound infiltration at Cesarean delivery for postoperative analgesia. *J Anesth*. 2013;27(2):175–179. doi: 10.1007/s00540-012-1510-7.

6. Bari MS, Haque N, Talukder SA, et al. Comparison of post operative pain relief between paracetamol and wound infiltration with levobupivacaine in inguinal hernia repair. *Mymensingh Med J*. 2012;21(3):411–415.

7. Jha AK, Bhardwaj N, Yaddanapudi S, et al. A randomized study of surgical site infiltration with bupivacaine or ketamine for pain relief in children following cleft palate repair. *Paediatr Anaesth*. 2013;23(5):401–406. doi: 10.1111/pan.12124.

8. Albi-Feldzer A, Mouret-Fourme EE, Hamouda S, et al. A double-blind randomized trial of wound and intercostals space infiltration with ropivacine during breast cancer surgery: effects on chronic postoperative pain. *Anesthesiology*. 2013;118(2):318–26. doi:10.1097/ALN.0b013e31827d88d8.

9. Chow TL, Choi CY, Lam SH. Parotidectomy under local anesthesia-report of 7 cases. *Am J Otolaryngol*. 2013;34(1):79–81. doi: 10.1016/j.amjoto.2012.08.012.

10. Budenz AW. Local anesthetics and medically complex patients. *J Calif Dent Assoc*. 2000;28(8):611–619.

11. Domingo DL, Canaan TJ. Local anesthetics (part II): assessment of adverse reactions and drug interactions. *Clinical Update*. 2002;24(10):20–22.

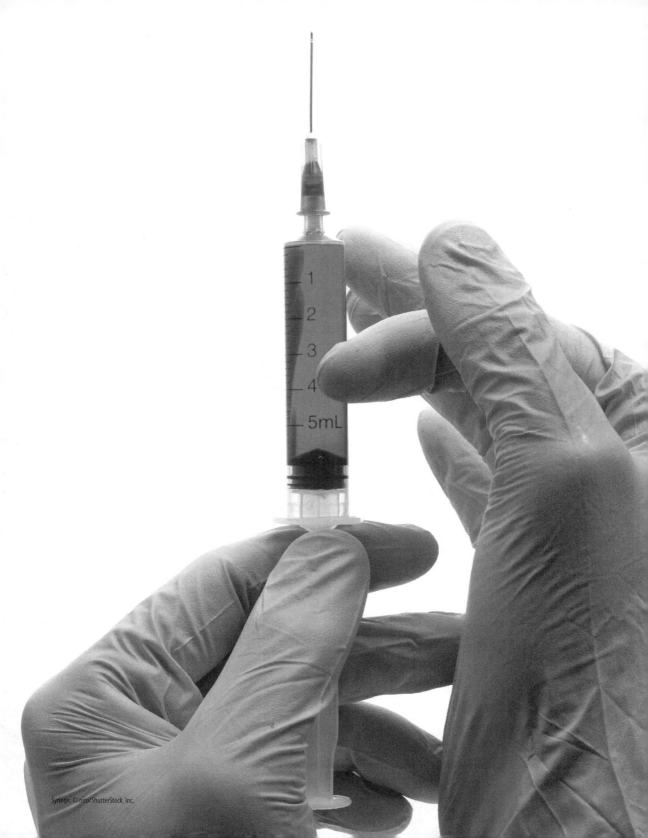

Syringe; © nito/ShutterStock, Inc.

CHAPTER 14

Dermatologic Procedures: Cryotherapy and Nail Biopsy

Abby Jacobson, MS, PA-C

PART I: CRYOTHERAPY

GOAL

▶ Utilize an extremely cold liquid or instrument on a targeted growth to freeze and destroy abnormal skin cells while leaving the surrounding skin free from injury.

OBJECTIVE

• Understand the indications for and procedure of cryotherapy, alternatives to cryotherapy, and the side effects of cryotherapy.

PART II: NAIL BIOPSY

GOALS

▶ Treat recalcitrant infections.
▶ Excise tumors of the nail unit.
▶ Allow full examination and exploration of the nail bed.
▶ Decrease the likelihood of chronic, painful nail plate deformity.

OBJECTIVE

• Understand the indications, procedure, and possible side effects of a nail biopsy.

PART I: CRYOTHERAPY

Rationale

- The general rationales for cryotherapy include its ease of use, its low cost, and its good cosmetic results. Cryosurgery is versatile, cost effective, and has advantages for patients who are allergic to local anesthesia or who take anticoagulants. Cryosurgery fits easily into the provider's schedule, requires no patient preparation, carries low risk of infection, and requires minimal wound care.

Evidence-Based Indications

- Cryotherapy is also known as liquid nitrogen cryosurgery. Utilization of cold in various forms can be traced back to the Egyptians of 2500 B.C.[1] While various substances have been used, liquid nitrogen is the current standard of care in cryotherapy. Cryotherapy involves the application of liquid nitrogen to the skin, causing direct injury to the cells and subsequent cell death.
- Removal of a benign lesion that negatively impacts activities of daily living (e.g., a **seborrheic keratosis** that is rubbing on clothing). It is essential to remember that cryotherapy destroys the tissue so there will be no ability for a pathology sample and subsequent pathology report. If there is any index of suspension of malignancy, cryotherapy should *not* be utilized and a biopsy should be performed to send all of the removed tissue for pathological analysis.
- Removal of viral lesions (e.g., verruca, *Molluscum contagiosum*).
- Removal of precancerous lesions known as **actinic keratoses** (AK).

Contraindications

- Concern for malignancy (see previous section).
- Risk of scarring may outweigh the benefits of removal of the lesion. Keloids or hypertrophic scars can develop from cryotherapy even when performed perfectly.
- Hyper- or hypopigmentation is a common side effect of cryotherapy. Most times the pigment will not normalize, even with time. Hypopigmentation in darker skin types (such as **Fitzpatrick skin types** IV, V, and VI) are at highest risk. For example, an African American patient with Fitzpatrick skin type V with papulosa nigra across the cheeks would most likely not benefit from cryotherapy because the hypopigmented scars would outweigh the benefit of their removal.
- Cryosurgery is uncomfortable to painful. Pain is perceived from a patient's perspective, with each person's perception of pain being unique to his or her experiences. This is important to take into account, especially in the pediatric population.

Complications

- Blister formation
- Bleeding (rare and minimal)
- Headache
- Hair loss
- Hypopigmentation
- Hyperpigmentation
- Scarring
- Procedural pain
- Residual and recurrent lesion
- Lesions that may require more than one treatment

Special Considerations

- Scarring, tolerability of the procedure, concerns of malignancy, and whether benefits outweigh risks.
- Factors determining the extent of cryogenic injury: choice of the cryogen, method of use and technique, freeze–thaw duration, efficiency of heat transfer, induced tissue ischemia, blood supply to the tissue, extent of vascular stasis after freezing.
- Anesthesia: Some patients may have a very low pain threshold. Others may report no

pain or sensation. Many patients will describe a burning sensation that lasts a few seconds, and burning usually stops quickly because the cryogen becomes its own anesthetic. Use of 1–2% lidocaine should be considered in sensitive or overly anxious patients. Remember to wait 5 minutes after injecting the lidocaine. Anesthetic spray or cream may be sprayed onto the treatment area prior to cryosurgery. Topical anesthetic cream such as topical lidocaine can take up to 1 hour to take effect. Therefore, with proper patient instruction, it can be applied at home prior to the procedure.

Supplies

- Liquid nitrogen. This can be applied to the skin either with a Q-tip or one of the many available handheld units (e.g., Brymill Cry-Ac units, Nitrograpy, Verruca-Freeze and Wallach UltraFreeze). See **FIGURE 14-1**.

FIGURE 14-1: Prepare supplies

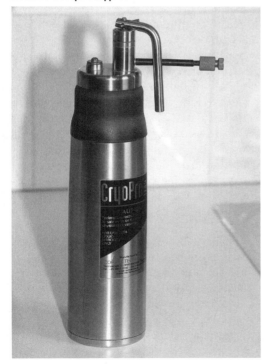

Procedural Instructions

- Patient preparation: Obtain consent.
- Non-sterile latex or vinyl exam gloves should be donned to protect the provider from some occasional mist or splattering of the cryogenic agent.
- To ease discomfort, some patients can apply topical anesthesia prior to the procedure (such as topical lidocaine). These topical agents will take time to take effect and should be used cautiously in the pediatric population.
- Select appropriate cone, extender tip, or tube to the cryotherapy apparatus and tank depending on the unit utilized.
- Apply liquid nitrogen via delivery system according to equipment instructions and type of lesion to be treated, being careful to avoid dripping of liquid nitrogen.
- The treated area will turn white, and patient may briefly feel slight tingling or burning sensation.
- Length of application of liquid nitrogen to the skin depends on patient tolerance, diagnosis of the lesion, size and depth of the lesion, and skin type. Temperatures of –25°C to –50°C (–13°F to –58°F) can be achieved within 30 seconds if a sufficient amount of liquid nitrogen is applied by spray or probe.[2] Repeated, shorter applications of liquid nitrogen are more effective than prolonged, direct application (see **TABLE 14-1**).[3] Margins for most benign lesions can extend as little as

TABLE 14-1: Suggested Length of Application of Liquid Nitrogen Based on Condition

Diagnosis	Length of Application
Actinic keratosis	5–10 seconds
Seborrheic keratosis	8–15 seconds
Verruca	8–20 seconds
Acrochordons	5 seconds

1 to 2 mm beyond the visible pathologic border. Premalignant lesions need margins of 2 to 3 mm.[2]

There are three general approaches to application:

1. Direct spray or application
2. Paintbrush technique
3. Spiral spraying

- After thawing, normal skin color returns and redness appears in the treated area 45–60 minutes after treatment. A blister or edema may form 24–48 hours post-treatment, and the treated area will change appearance over the next few days and will slough off in 7–14 days.

Post-procedure Instructions

- No dressing is necessary immediately after freezing. If the bullous formation begins draining in 2–3 days, a small gauze pad covering might be beneficial for 1–2 days.
- Leave the lesion uncovered at night to facilitate healing.
- Cleansing the lesion may be indicated in the initial 3–5 days post-treatment.

PART II: NAIL BIOPSY

Rationale for Procedure

- A nail biopsy is a surgical technique to gain a diagnosis of ambiguous nail disorders. This surgical procedure is indicated after a complete medical and clinical history fails to diagnose the condition. Nail surgical procedures are most frequently performed by dermatologists, dermatologic surgeons, orthopedic surgeons, and plastic surgeons of the hand. It can be performed with minimal pain and scarring and without permanent dystrophy. A variety of nail biopsy techniques are reviewed in this chapter. The essentials of a successful nail biopsy begin with an understanding of nail anatomy, blood supply to the nail, hemostasis, nerves, and anesthesia.

- A thorough understanding of the anatomy of the nail unit is essential for a successful nail biopsy. The nail unit consists of the proximal nail fold (PNF), matrix, nail bed, and hyponychium. The PNF is a fold of skin of the dorsal aspect of the distal digit. The nail plate arises from under the PNF. The epithelium of the ventral surface of the PNF is also known as the eponychium. The nail matrix forms the floor of the nail bed. It is visible as the half-moon-shaped structure at the base of the nail known as the lunula. The matrix forms the nail plate. Damage to the matrix of the nail unit can cause permanent scarring. The nail bed ends beneath the nail plate at the beginning of the hyponychium. The hyponychium represents the beginning of normal epidermis distal to the end of the nail bed.

Evidence-Based Indications

- The most frequent indications to sample a nail unit are tumors. Nail tumors include melanoma, squamous cell carcinoma, **pyogenic granuloma**, and osteochondroma. Inflammatory nail diseases such as functional melanonychia, lichen planus, psoriasis, and **onychomycosis** are also indications for a nail biopsy. Melanoma is by far the most deadly. The prognosis is poor, ranging from 16–87% 5-year survival. This is due to a delayed diagnosis and the fact that nail melanoma is more aggressive than most cutaneous melanomas. The thumb and the big toe are most frequently affected.

Types of Nail Biopsies

- The most common types of nail biopsies include punch biopsy, excisional biopsy, and longitudinal biopsy. The type of biopsy chosen depends on the site within the nail unit. An excisional biopsy is preferred over a punch biopsy, especially if melanoma is in the differential diagnosis. Also, it is important to properly orient the excision. An excision in the nail bed is oriented longitudinally, while the nail matrix excision is oriented horizontally. Special instruments are utilized in nail surgeries. The Freer septum elevator is used to avulse the nail while protecting the matrix. Dual-action nail clippers easily remove portions of the nail for easy exposure.

- *Punch biopsy.* The histopathology is often challenging in the case of a small 3-mm punch biopsy through the nail because only a small sampling of the nail matrix is achieved with this type of biopsy. A 3-mm punch biopsy leaves a minimal scar and no suturing is necessary. A punch biopsy is useful to sample the nail plate when a proximal white onychomycosis is suspected.
- *Excisional biopsy.* The nail is avulsed prior to removing the specimen. The excision should be oriented along the longitudinal axis and the excision should be elliptical. Defects larger than 3 mm should be sutured.
- *Longitudinal biopsy.* The nail is avulsed, and an excision is performed deep to the bone. The defect is closed with absorbable suture material. This is often used to diagnose longitudinal melanonychia. There is a higher risk for splitting of the nail, especially when the proximal or mid-matrix is affected.

Complications

- Complications include infection, hematoma, and nail deformity.
- Careful patient selection should be considered before performing a nail biopsy. Patients at higher risk for infection should be selected and preoperatively treated with antibiotics. Infection of the nail unit is uncommon due to the vasculature of the digits.
- Sterile technique and preparation of the skin and nail prior to the procedure are important. Achieving hemostasis in any procedure at risk for bleeding minimizes the risk of developing hematomas.
- Nail deformity is the result of nail matrix damage. Gentle care of the nail matrix and

an understanding of the nail unit anatomy is necessary in achieving good postoperative results.

Procedural Instructions

- Patient consent is obtained with careful explanation of future potential nail deformity.
- The extremity is cleansed with a surgical cleansing agent.
- A sterile surgical field must be maintained throughout the procedure.
- Local anesthetic is used with nail biopsy. This is injected locally or more often by digital block—when the anesthetic is injected through the web spaces along each side of the finger or toe. The cutaneous sensory nerves run parallel to the blood vessels along the lateral digit. There are three main types of distal digital anesthesia required for a nail biopsy. One is a distal digital block, also known as the wing block, which offers a total unit anesthesia. A needle with 2 mL of plain lidocaine is injected 2–3 mm proximal to the junction of the proximal and lateral nail fold. The opposite side is also anesthetized in the same manner. The second type is the distal anesthesia through the proximal nail fold. The needle with 0.5 to 1 mL of plain lidocaine is injected very slowly into the middle of the PNF. The lunula and nail bed will begin to blanch. The third type of nail block is the distal anesthesia through the hyponychium. This is more painful for the patient and therefore is not performed very often. The needle with plain lidocaine is inserted into the lateral hyponychium and directed horizontally in the nail bed while the lidocaine is injected (see **FIGURE 14-2**).
- A wide Penrose drain is used for hemostasis.
- The nail plate may be completely avulsed for biopsy, but complete avulsion is not always indicated. A partial avulsion of the proximal one-third of the plate may be performed, leaving the distal two-thirds of the nail plate intact.

FIGURE 14-2: Anesthetize affected area

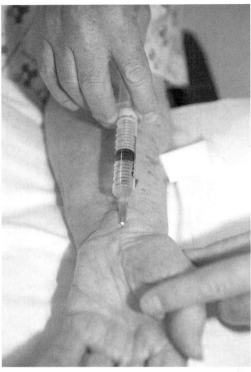

© Dr. P. Marazzi/Science Source

- After avulsion, the matrix is exposed.
- Next, biopsy of the matrix can be performed.
- Hemostasis can be achieved by applying manual pressure to the lateral digital arteries during the procedures. Another method is to use a tourniquet with a flat Penrose drain. If a tourniquet is used, it is important to remove after 15 minutes.
- Following the procedure, keep nail clean and dry.

▶ **REFERENCES**

1. Squazzi A, Bracco D. A historical count of the technical means used in cryotherapy. *Minerva Med.* 1974;65:3718.

2. Andrews MD. Cryosurgery for common skin conditions. *Am Fam Physician.* 2004; 69(10):2365–2372.

3. Freedberg IM, Fitzpatrick TB. *Fitzpatrick's Dermatology in General Medicine.* 6th ed. New York, NY: McGraw-Hill; 2003: 2575–2581.

▶ **ADDITIONAL READING**

Collins CC, Cordova BK, Jellinek JN. Midline/paramedian longitudinal matrix excision with flap reconstruction: alternative surgical techniques for evaluation of longitudinal melanonychia. *J Am Acad Dermatol.* 2010;64(4):627–636.

Moossavi M, Scher KR. Complications of nail surgery: a review of the literature. *Dermatol Surg.* 2001;27(3):225–228.

Rich P. Nail biopsy: indications and methods. *Dermatol Surg.* 2001;27(3):229–234.

Scher KR, Daniel RC, III. *Nails: Diagnosis, Therapy and Surgery.* 3rd ed. New York, NY: Elsevier Saunders; 2005.

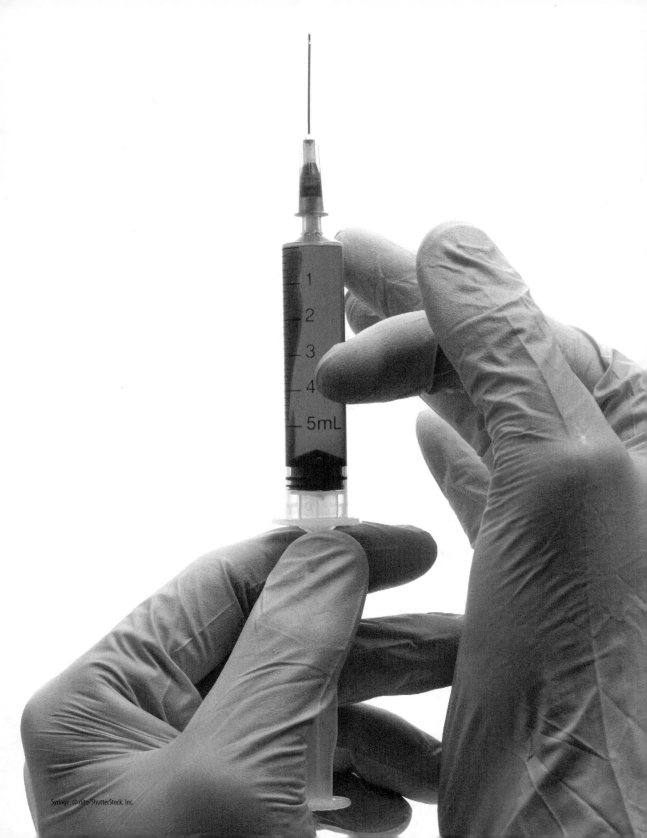

CHAPTER 15

Gynecology: Cervical Cancer Screening

Nina Multak, MPAS, PA-C

GOAL

▶ Reduce the incidence of cases and deaths from cervical cancer.

OBJECTIVES

1. Understand the procedure for the Pap smear.
2. Identify the techniques for obtaining a Pap smear.
3. Gain familiarity with the reporting system.

RATIONALE FOR PROCEDURE

- Cervical cancer screening can detect very early changes that, untreated, could lead to invasive cervical disease. Pap smear screening practices, the role of human papillomavirus (HPV) testing, and development of new technologies have contributed to continuous reevaluation of cervical cancer screening practices. An extended time period between the detection of abnormalities by screening and the development of invasive cancer incites continuous reevaluation of appropriate frequency of testing.

EVIDENCE-BASED INDICATIONS

- The United States Preventive Services Task Force (USPSTF) and the American Cancer Society (ACS) currently advise that cervical cytology screening in women should begin at age 21 years, with less frequent subsequent rescreening than suggested in its earlier guidelines.[1] Women ages 21–29 should receive cervical cancer screening once every 3 years. Screening using either the conventional Pap or the liquid-based method is acceptable.
- For women ages 30–65 years who have had negative Pap test results, the recommended screening strategy includes co-testing with the Pap test (using the conventional Pap or liquid-based method) combined with HPV testing once every 5 years. A Pap test alone (without HPV co-testing) once every 3 years is acceptable for women in this age group if HPV testing is not available.
- Cervical cancer screening should be discontinued in women over 65 years of age if they have no history of cervical intraepithelial neoplasia (CIN 2), CIN 3, adenocarcinoma *in situ*, or cervical cancer, and who have also had either 3 consecutive negative Pap test results or 2 consecutive negative co-test (Pap and HPV) results within the previous 10 years, with the most recent test performed within the past 5 years. Women who have had a hysterectomy with removal of the cervix and have no history of CIN 2 or CIN 3 can discontinue routine cervical cancer screening.

CONTRAINDICATIONS

- No absolute contraindications are known other than reasons for discontinuation already mentioned.

COMPLICATIONS

- Spotting and pelvic cramping may follow Pap smear sampling.
- Laboratory factors that diminish the accuracy of Pap smears include:
  - Failure to identify dysplastic cells
  - Misinterpretation of cells
  - Poorly utilized technical process
- Clinician factors that diminish the accuracy of Pap smears include:
  - Contamination with blood or oil-based lubricants
  - Mislabeled or unlabeled cell samples
  - Inadequate clinical history
  - Inadequate sampling of the transformation zone
  - Collected material too thick or insufficient
  - Presence of infection

SPECIAL CONSIDERATIONS

- Visual inspection of the lower genital tract and cervix through the speculum by the clinician enables optimal sample collection.
- An optimal cervical specimen includes sampling of the squamous and columnar epithelium, including the transformation zone, where the majority of cervical neoplasias arise.
- The location and appearance of the transformation zone may vary depending on such factors as vaginal pH, pregnancy, age, prior medications, and individual anatomy.

SUPPLIES

- Non-sterile gloves
- Speculums of various sizes and types (Pedersen, Graves; see **FIGURES 15-1** and **15-2**)
- A light source
- Water-soluble lubricant
- Large swabs for gentle blotting of excess discharge
- Wooden spatulas or plastic spatulas for ectocervical sample
- Cytobrush for endocervical sample
- A "broom" device, which can be used for ectodermal and endocervical samples
- Microscope slides and fixative or cytology preservative solution for liquid-based testing

FIGURE 15-1: Gynecological speculum

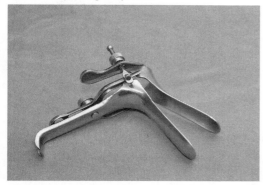

© Praisaeng/ShutterStock, Inc.

FIGURE 15-2: Plastic speculum

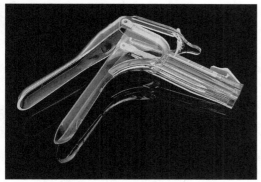

© Elizabeth Dover/ShutterStock, Inc.

PROCEDURAL INSTRUCTIONS

- Obtain informed consent.
- Wash your hands and prepare gloves.
- Instruct the patient about exam contents as the exam proceeds to ease anxiousness.
- Position the patient: Place the patient in a supine position on the exam table with her heels in the stirrups and with her buttocks just at the edge or just over the edge of the exam table to facilitate speculum insertion.
- Draping: Draping should be used to protect the patients modesty and help make the patient more comfortable. The drape should be moved or adjusted to enable the clinician to appropriately perform the procedure.
- Lighting: Good lighting is important and is often accomplished with a goose-neck lamp.
- Cover foot rests: Use a protective cover to warm and cushion the stirrups.
- Inspect the vulva: Gently spread the labia apart and inspect the vulva, moving the labia and skin folds, inspecting for:
  - Skin lesions
  - Masses
  - Drainage
  - Discolorations of the skin
  - Signs of trauma
  - Pubic hair distribution

Inserting the Speculum

- After warming the speculum (see **FIGURE 15-3**), separate the labia and keep them apart.

FIGURE 15-3: Select appropriate speculum

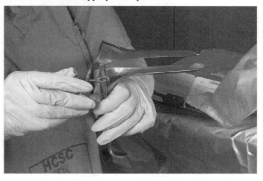

FIGURE 15-4: Insert speculum at oblique angle

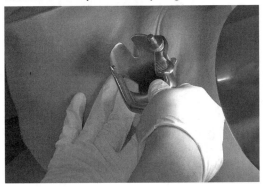

FIGURE 15-5: Visualize the cervix

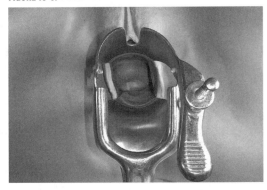

FIGURE 15-6: Impact of cervical cancer—normal and abnormal cervixes

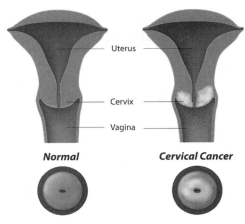

© Alila Sao Mai/ShutterStock, Inc.

- Insert the speculum into the vagina (see **FIGURE 15-4**). Keep the speculum blades closed until the speculum is completely inserted.
- Open the speculum; usually, the cervix is immediately visible. If not, gently moving the speculum inferiorly or superiorly in small movements will usually allow the cervix to come into view.
- Lock the blades in the open position, wide enough apart to allow complete visualization of the cervix (see **FIGURE 15-5**).

Collecting the Pap Smear

Preparation to Collect Pap Smear—Speculum Insertion and Visualization

- Label the sample container for a liquid-based Pap smear or the end of the glass slide with the patient's name prior to sample collection. Some liquid-based Pap tests have the advantage of additional tests being ordered and run from the same sample (i.e., HPV, chlamydia, gonorrhea).
- Insert the speculum, which may be moistened with water or saline if necessary.
  - A heating pad may be used to keep the speculums warm.
  - Lubricants are not recommended because they may interfere with interpretation of the results.
- Visually inspect the cervix for abnormalities (see **FIGURE 15-6**).
- Identify the **transformation zone**.
  - The endocervical limit of the transformation zone is dynamic, defined by the leading edge of the migrating squamocolumnar junction.
  - In postmenopausal women, it is often high in the endocervical canal and not visible.

Collecting the Pap Smear—Spatula

- Choose the contoured, concave end of the spatula, which fits best across the cervix and the transformation zone (see **FIGURE 15-7**).

FIGURE 15-7: **Obtain cervical specimen using spatula (cervix model)**

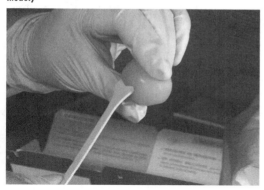

- Rotate the spatula 360° on the circumference of the cervix, while maintaining contact with the epithelial surface (see FIGURE 15-8).
- With a clockwise rotation beginning and ending at 9 o'clock (or counterclockwise rotation from 3 o'clock to 3 o'clock), the collected cellular sample is retained on the upper horizontal surface as the spatula is removed.
- Hold the spatula with the non-sampling hand while the cervical brush sample is collected.
- Spread the sample collected on the spatula evenly over the slide with a single smooth movement or place into specified liquid-based cytology container.

Collecting the Pap Smear—Cervix Brush

- These brushes have circumferential bristles that come into contact with the entire os surface on insertion.
- The brush should be rotated (see FIGURE 15-9).
- Roll the brush across the slide by twirling the handle (see FIGURE 15-10).
  - If using a slide, the objective is to quickly and evenly spread the cellular sample in a single layer on the slide.
  - Transfer material from both sampling instruments to the slide within a few seconds and fix immediately in order to avoid air-drying artifact.
  - Immediately fix the specimen by either immersing the slide into the specified container or covering the slide with a surface fixative.

Spatula and Brush—Options for Transferring Sample

- Option 1:
  - Smear the spatula on the upper half of the slide (see FIGURE 15-11).
  - Roll the brush across the lower half of the slide.
  - Immediately fix slide.

FIGURE 15-8: **Use spatula to obtain cervical specimens**

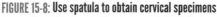
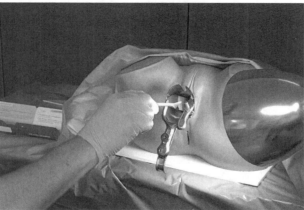

FIGURE 15-9: Use cervical brush in endocervix

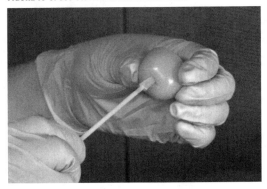

FIGURE 15-10: Rotate the cervical specimen

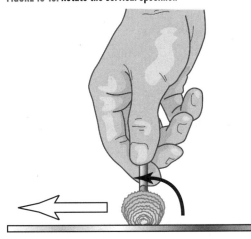

FIGURE 15-11: Obtain cervical cell samples

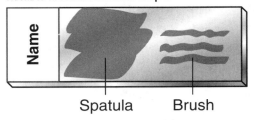

- Option 2:
  - Smear the spatula sample over the left-hand side of the slide, cover the righthand side with cardboard, and immediately spray fixative.

FIGURE 15-12: Application of cervical cells to slide

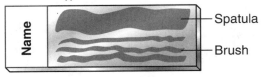

- Roll the brush material onto the right-hand side of the slide and use fixative (see **FIGURE 15-12**).

Collecting the Pap Smear—Plastic "Broom"

- Another collection instrument is a plastic broom-like brush that samples the **endocervix** and **ectocervix**.
- To use the broom, insert the long central bristles into the cervical os until the lateral bristles bend against the ectocervix. Rotate 3–5 times in both directions.
  - To transfer material, smear both sides of the broom across the glass slide. Place the second stroke exactly over the first stroke (see **FIGURE 15-13**).
- In a liquid-based Pap cytology test, cervical cells collected with a brush or other instrument are placed in a vial of liquid preservative. The slide or vial is then sent to a laboratory for evaluation.
- A bimanual pelvic exam usually follows the collection of the two samples for the Pap smear. The bimanual examination involves the healthcare practitioner inserting 2 gloved fingers of 1 hand inside the vaginal canal while palpating the ovaries, adnexa, and uterus with the other hand on top of the abdomen.

FIGURE 15-13: Apply cervical specimen

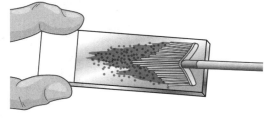

REPORTING SYSTEM: INTERPRETATION OF RESULTS[2]

The following information comes from the National Cancer Institute (2014).

- The *Bethesda System* is a uniform nomenclature for Pap smear cytology interpretation. The Pap smear report should indicate whether the smear was adequate. Unless the patient has had a hysterectomy, the report should include cytologic evidence that the transformation zone was sampled.

- *Negative for intraepithelial lesion or malignancy.* Samples that are normal have no cell abnormalities (see **FIGURE 15-14**). A negative Pap test report may also indicate non-neoplastic findings (e.g., infections or inflammation).

- *Atypical squamous cells (ASC)* are the most common abnormal finding in Pap tests. The Bethesda System divides this category into the following two groups:
  - *ASC-US*: Atypical squamous cells of undetermined significance. The squamous cells do not appear completely normal, but there is uncertainty about what the cell changes mean. Sometimes the changes are related to an HPV infection, but they can also be caused by other factors. For women who have ASC-US, a sample of cells may be tested for the presence of high-risk HPV types.
  - *ASC-H*: Atypical squamous cells; cannot exclude a high-grade squamous intraepithelial lesion. The cells do not appear normal, but there is uncertainty about what the cell changes mean. ASC-H lesions may be at higher risk of being precancerous compared with ASC-US lesions.

- *Low-grade squamous intraepithelial lesions (LSILs)* are considered mild abnormalities caused by HPV infection. "Low-grade" means that there are early changes in the size and shape of cells. LSILs are sometimes classified as mild dysplasia. LSILs can also be classified as cervical intraepithelial neoplasia (CIN-1).

- *High-grade squamous intraepithelial lesions (HSILs)* are more severe abnormalities that have a higher likelihood of progressing to cancer if left untreated. High-grade means that there are more evident changes in the size and shape of the abnormal (precancerous) cells and that the cells look very different from normal cells. HSILs include lesions with moderate or severe dysplasia and carcinoma

FIGURE 15-14: Normal cervix

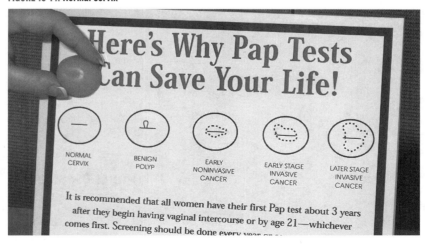

FIGURE 15-15: Invasive cancer

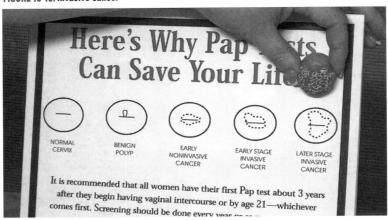

in situ (CIS). HSIL lesions are sometimes classified as CIN-2, CIN-3, or CIN-2/3. CIS is commonly included in the CIN-3 category.

- *Squamous cell carcinoma* is cervical cancer. The abnormal squamous cells have invaded deeper into the cervix or into other tissues or organs (see **FIGURE 15-15**).
- *Atypical glandular cells (AGC)* imply that the glandular cells do not appear normal, but there is uncertainty about the interpretation of this finding.
- *Endocervical adenocarcinoma in situ (AIS)* means that precancerous cells are found only in tissue of the cervix.
- *Adenocarcinoma* includes cancer of the endocervical canal and, in some patients, endometrial, extrauterine, and other cancers.

AFTERCARE INSTRUCTIONS

- The American Society for Colposcopy and Cervical Pathology (ASCCP) developed guidelines for the management of abnormal cervical cytology.[3] The ASCCP guidelines are summarized with algorithms that can guide clinicians through evidence-based recommendations for most abnormal Pap smear scenarios.
- A report that describes glandular or adenomatous atypia warrants immediate colposcopy with endocervical curettage to rule out a high-grade lesion and cervical adenocarcinoma. If the findings of AGC are definite, cone biopsy, pelvic ultrasound, and laparoscopy may be indicated.

▶ REFERENCES

1. Committee on Practice Bulletins—Gynecology. ACOG practice bulletin number 131: screening for cervical cancer. *Obstet Gynecol.* 2012;120(5):1222–1238.
2. National Cancer Institute. *PAP and HPV Testing.* National Institutes of Health. http://www.cancer.gov/cancertopics/factsheet/detection/Pap-HPV-testing. September 9, 2014. Accessed July 9, 2015.
3. Saslow D, Solomon D, Lawson HW, et al. American Cancer Society, American Society for Colposcopy and Cervical Pathology, and American Society for Clinical Pathology screening guidelines for the prevention and early detection of cervical cancer. *CA Cancer J Clin.* 2012;62(3):147–172.

▶ ADDITIONAL READING

Hughey M. OBGYN 101. Brookside Associates. http://www.brooksidepress.org/Products/OBGYN_101/. Accessed July 9, 2015.

UNIT 2

ADVANCED PROCEDURES

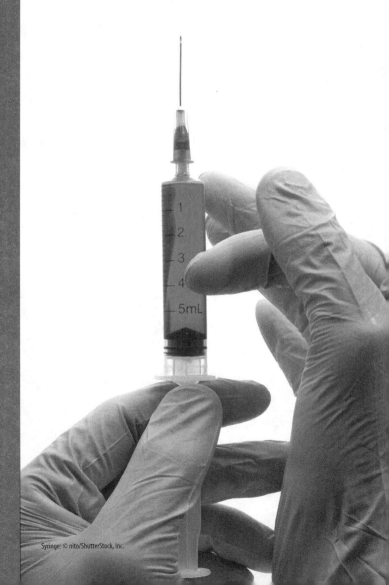

Syringe: © nito/ShutterStock, Inc.

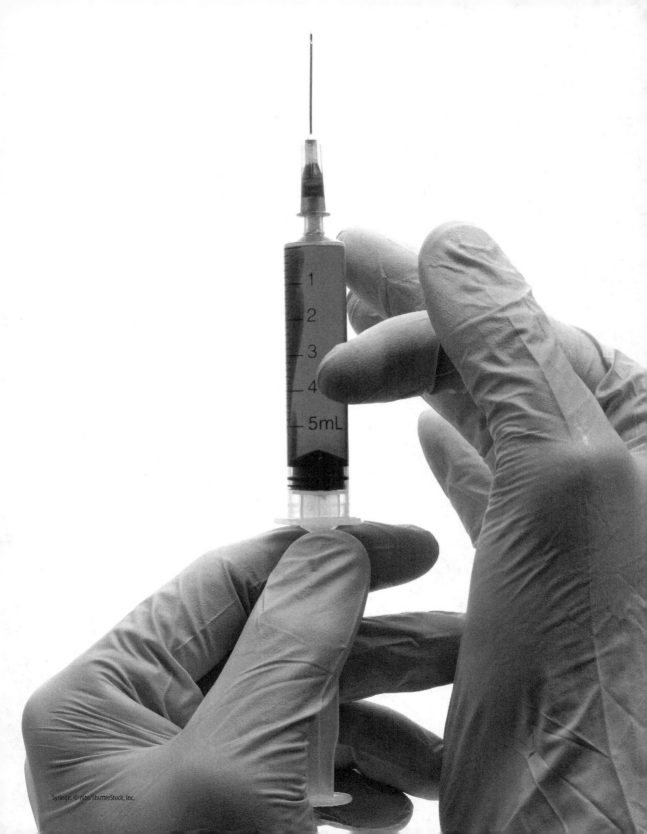

CHAPTER 16
Chest Tube Insertion and Removal

Jim Burkett, MS, EMT-P, PA-C

GOALS

▶ Drain abnormal collections of fluid from the pleural cavity.

▶ Treat spontaneous or traumatic pnuemothorax.

OBJECTIVES

1. Gain the knowledge and skills to effectively place and remove a chest tube, also known as a tube thoracostomy.
2. Describe the indications and contraindications of tube thoracostomy.
3. Recognize the potential complications of tube thoracostomy placement and removal as well as prevention and treatment.
4. Consider the major indications and discuss site placement and equipment selection.
5. Describe the setup and operation of suction, valves, and drainage systems.
6. Demonstrate the proper use of protective barriers and site preparation used during placement and removal.
7. Describe proper patient positioning and anesthesia.
8. Describe tube placement, securing, and dressings.
9. Understand the steps for tube removal.
10. Describe follow-up care and patient education.

RATIONALE FOR PROCEDURE

- As is the case for most of emergency medicine, the origin of tube thoracostomy was military medical care.[1] Toward the end of World War I, the use of chest tubes began to gain acceptance, and during World War II, the U.S. Army Medical Department published treatment guidelines for the management of tension pneumothorax and for chest tube drainage.[2]
- Closed thoracostomy has been the standard of care for the emergency treatment of pneumothorax and hemothorax.
- The alternative treatment is an open thoracostomy, which requires additional time, training, and resources and has more severe negative consequences for the patient.

EVIDENCED-BASED INDICATIONS

- A chest tube is needed when there is a disruption of the normal chest pathophysiology. The integrity of the system is disrupted by the collection of air, blood, or fluid in the pleural space, which leads to lung collapse and compromises respiration. A tube thoracostomy evacuates these abnormal collections as a specific treatment modality.
- Chest tubes may also be placed to aid in diagnosis, or as a temporizing measure, until definitive treatment is initiated. Additionally, chest tubes may be used during an open thoracotomy to aid in postoperative recovery and monitoring of the patient.
- The common indications for chest tube placement are:
  - **Pneumothorax**; open or closed, simple or tension
  - **Hemothorax**
  - **Hemopneumothorax**
  - **Hydrothorax**
  - **Chylothorax**
  - **Empyema**
  - Pleural effusion

- Penetrating chest injuries requiring intubation
- Postoperative thoracotomy treatment

CONTRAINDICATIONS
Absolute Contraindication

- A 2007 article, published in the *New England Journal of Medicine*, stated the only absolute contraindication for a chest tube is when the lung is completely adherent with the hemothorax.[3] If an open thoracotomy is emergent, a chest tube should not be placed if it would delay the open procedure.

Relative Contraindications

- Significant coagulopathy
- Pulmonary bullae
- Pleura adhesions
- Skin infection at the insertion site

COMPLICATIONS OF PLACEMENT

- A major complication during placement is bleeding from intercostal or major vessels; another major complication is inadvertent injury to visceral organs, causing a life-threatening hemorrhage or a delayed, slow bleeding from improper placement.
- Subcutaneous emphysema is a complication that may develop if the tube is dislodged or if one of the chest tube side holes is withdrawn into the chest wall tissues. Persistent bubbling indicating an air leak in the water seal drainage system may identify this complication.
- The most common complication, which should be mentioned specifically on the consent form, is intercostal neuralgia. This complication occurs either from direct neurovascular damage during placement or from irritation to the costal nerves while the tube is in place. Intercostal neuralgia is extremely uncomfortable and must be considered

if the patient is experiencing pain at the chest wall puncture site or in the placement dermatome.

- Four problem areas of significant importance were identified in a video analysis of 50 chest tube insertions that affect the provider or the patient.[4] These parts of the procedure should be given special attention in order to avoid complications: breaks in sterile technique, inadequate anesthesia, incorrect insertion technique, and inadequate self-protection.

SPECIAL CONSIDERATIONS

- In certain clinical scenarios, only an experienced individual should perform the tube thoracostomy. These cases include patients on ventilators, patients who require multiple chest tubes, patients with adhesions, or patients with chronic lung disease. Tube thoracostomies under these clinical conditions are not discussed here.

SUPPLIES

- Before starting the tube thoracostomy, equipment should be set up on a stand in the order in which it will be used.
- A water seal drainage system, such as the Pleur-evac, should be prepared prior to the procedure. Each chest drainage system has specific setup requirements; therefore, the appropriate user manual should be referenced.
- Lidocaine 1% with epinephrine
- Syringes, 10–20 mL (2)
- Needle, 25 gauge (ga), ⅝ inch (in)
- Needle, 23 ga, 1.5 in; or 27 ga, 1.5 in; for instilling local anesthesia
- Blade, No. 10, on a handle
- Large and medium Kelly clamps
- Large curved Mayo scissors
- Large straight suture scissors
- Suture, 0 or 1-0
- Needle driver

- Gauze squares, 4 × 4 in (10)
- Sterile adhesive tape, 4 in wide
- Chest tube of appropriate size
  - Man: 28–32 French (Fr)
  - Woman: 28 Fr
  - Child: 12–28 Fr
  - Infant: 12–16 Fr

PROCEDURAL INSTRUCTIONS: CHEST TUBE INSERTION

- As with any procedure, the provider should begin with the patient consent form. In a non-life-threatening emergency, this is a requirement that facilitates the procedure. The consent process informs the patient and family of what will occur and provides an opportunity for positive patient identification.
- The patient should be positioned for comfort and for optimal access to the insertion site.
- With the patient supine, the bed should be slightly elevated to 30°–45°.
- In order to improve exposure, place a pillow under the patient on the procedure side to elevate the lateral chest wall off the bed.
- The arm on the affected side should be raised over the head to a comfortable position.
- Using maximum sterile universal barrier precautions (handwashing, head cover, facemask with eye protection, sterile gown, and sterile gloves), create a large surgical field at the insertion site using a skin-prep solution of chlorhexidine or povidone-iodine (Betadine).
- Use large sterile drapes exposing only the insertion site.
- The insertion site selection should be within the area known as the "Triangle of Safety."[5] This area corresponds to the anterior border of the latissimus dorsi, the lateral border of the pectoralis major, and the apex just below the axilla in a horizontal line with the nipple (see **FIGURE 16-1**).

FIGURE 16-1: Anatomic landmarks

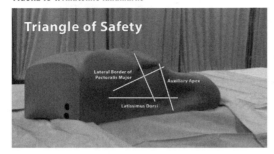

FIGURE 16-2: Anesthetize insertion area

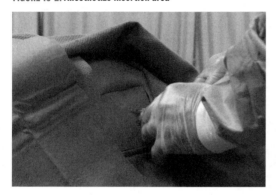

FIGURE 16-3A: Blunt dissection

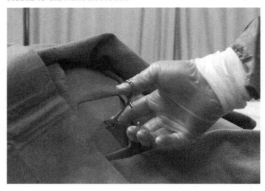

FIGURE 16-3B: Kelly forceps for blunt dissection

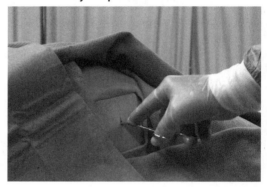

- Palpating the 5th rib, inject a local anesthetic of lidocaine or bupivacaine (Marcaine), creating a skin wheel at the insertion site with a 25-gauge, 1¼-inch needle (see **FIGURE 16-2**).
- Switch to a larger needle, such as a 21-gauge, to anesthetize the subcutaneous tissues and intercostal muscles along the planned tract.
- The periosteum over the 5th rib should also be anesthetized. Inadequate analgesia is frequently encountered during chest tube insertion. Therefore, consideration should be given to the use of a short-acting IV narcotic, such as fentanyl, to supplement the local anesthetic.
- Using a #10-scalpel blade, an approximately 2- to 3-cm transverse incision should be made.

- Bluntly dissect down over the rib; then, using large Kelly forceps, dissect superiorly over the rib through the intercostal muscles to the parietal pleura and gently push through into the pleural space (see **FIGURE 16-3**).
- When entering the pleura, both hands need to be used to maintain a controlled entry and avoid lung damage. Spread the forceps to enlarge the hole and tract. A rush of air and/or fluid should occur, verifying your location.
- If placing a larger chest tube, insert a gloved finger into the tract and pleural space to ensure there are no adhesions and no solid organs have been entered. In trauma cases involving possible rib fractures, be cautious in order to avoid punctures from sharp bone ends.

FIGURE 16-4: Insert chest tube

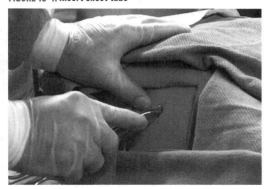

- Holding the fenestrated end of the chest tube with a Kelly clamp and having the opposite end of the chest tube crossed-clamped, insert the fenestrated end of the tube over a gloved finger or blindly through the tract (see **FIGURE 16-4**).
- Remove the clamp and gently guide the tube into position. The tip should be placed apically for a pneumothorax and posteriorly inferior for a fluid collection, making sure all of the fenestrated side holes are within the pleura space (see **FIGURE 16-5**).

- The tube should be secured using two O-silk simple sutures on each side of the tube. Wrap and tie the suture ends around the tube multiple times, using what is known as a Roman-sandal knot.
- To facilitate tube removal, place a horizontal mattress suture, but do not tie it in place. Instead, tie the end in an overhand knot and wrap it around the chest tube to keep the tube in place until removal.
- The chest tube is connected to the drainage system and the cross Kelly clamp is removed. This connection will need to be reinforced with either plastic cable ties or tape. Petroleum and a 4- × 4-inch gauze dressing should be placed around the base of the tube, and wide cloth tape should be applied, making an airtight seal (see **FIGURE 16-6**).
- The chest drainage system is initially set to −20 cm of water pressure and adjusted by protocol.
- After securing the chest tube and applying the dressing, the patient should be examined for complications.
- A portable chest x-ray must be taken to confirm proper placement, and the provider should review the x-ray.

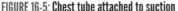

FIGURE 16-5: Chest tube attached to suction

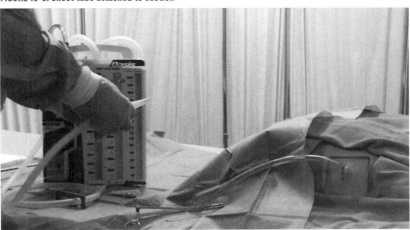

FIGURE 16-6: Secure tubing prior to dressing application

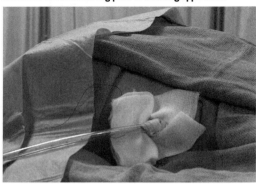

PROCEDURAL INSTRUCTIONS: CHEST TUBE REMOVAL

- When to remove the chest tube depends on the reason for its insertion. For a simple pneumothorax, bubbling should have ceased while on suction, the lung fully expanded, and the pulmonary clinical findings improved. A trial of being off suction, using only the water seal or clamping the tube to rule out a persistent air leak, is normally employed with a repeat chest x-ray 12–24 hours later.
- When removing the chest tube, the clinician may wish to assess whether removal should be done during end-inspiration or end-expiration. The clinical evidence on this suggests that it does not appear to matter.[6]
- Ideally, two people using sterile technique with patient and provider barrier protection should remove the tube. After cutting the ties around the tube, one provider would instruct the patient on breathing while pulling the tube, while a second would tie the suture that was placed on insertion to occlude the tube tract.
- Vaseline gauze and 4- × 4-inch dressings should be ready to be placed over the wound. One or two packets of O-suture should be immediately available in case the suture breaks while tying.

AFTERCARE INSTRUCTIONS

- The patient should be examined and another chest x-ray taken 12 to 24 hours after removal of the chest tube. The clinician should look for a reoccurrence of the pneumothorax or other complications, such as delayed bleeding.
- The patient and family should be given instructions on wound care, activity, and potential future complications.

► **REFERENCES**

1. Monaghan SF, Swan KG. Tube thoracostomy: the struggle to the "standard of care." *The Ann Thor Surg.* 2008;86(6):2019–2022.

2. General USPHS, Oot S, Berry FB, Coates JB, Dept USAM. *Surgery in World War II: Thoracic Surgery.* Washington, DC: Office of the Surgeon-General, Department of the Army; 1963.

3. Dev SP, Nascimiento Jr B, Simone C, Chien V. Chest-tube insertion. *N Engl J Med.* 2007;357(15):e15.

4. *Problems and Preventions: Chest Tube Insertion* [DVD]. Silver Springs, MD: Agency for Healthcare Research and Quality; 2006.

5. Laws D, Neville E, Duffy J. BTS guidelines for the insertion of a chest drain. *Thorax.* 2003;58(suppl 2):ii53–ii59.

6. Bell RL, Ovadia P, Abdullah F, Spector S, Rabinovici R. Chest tube removal: end-inspiration or end-expiration? *J Trauma.* 2001;50(4):674.

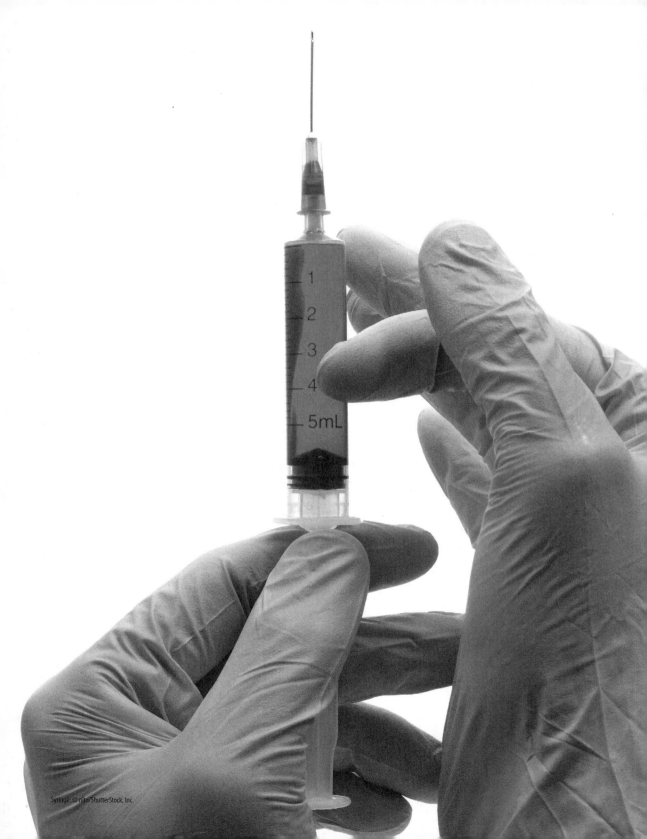

CHAPTER 17

Arterial Cannulation: Insertion and Removal

Poovendran Saththasivam, MD
Michael Green, DO

GOALS

▶ Monitor the hemodynamic status of critically ill patients.

▶ Arterial blood gas sampling.

OBJECTIVES

1. Identify the benefit of arterial cannulation.
2. Identify the most common artery used for monitoring blood pressure in critically ill patients.
3. Identify other common vessels cannulated for blood pressure monitoring.

RATIONALE FOR PROCEDURE

- Arterial cannulation is an invasive method of monitoring blood pressure in critically ill patients.
- The artery most commonly cannulated is the radial; however, the brachial, axillary, femoral, and dorsalis pedis arteries are other potential locations.
- Cannulation allows for beat-to-beat arterial blood pressure monitoring.
- Faster recognition of changes in hemodynamics is provided, which allows for adjustment of vasoactive drug infusion, frequent blood sampling, and determination of continuous cardiac output using pulse contour method.

EVIDENCE-BASED INDICATIONS

- Arterial catheters can be placed at the bedside and have been found to be relatively safe, with a low incidence of serious complications.
- An arterial catheter allows for continuous blood pressure monitoring, frequent blood sampling, and arterial blood gas measurement.
- The **radial artery** is most commonly used in both adults and children.
- Arterial cannulation is performed when frequent arterial blood gas analysis is indicated.

CONTRAINDICATIONS[1]

- Absolute contraindications are absence of pulse, Buerger disease, full-thickness burn over cannulation site, Raynaud's disease, and compromised circulation to extremity.
- Relative contraindications are patients on anticoagulation, atherosclerosis, coagulopathy, and presence of local skin infection.

COMPLICATIONS

- Complications from arterial cannulation are extremely rare, but providers must maintain vigilance in recognition due to the serious nature.

- Complications include arterial thrombosis leading to limb ischemia or gangrene, fistula formation, arterial dissection, hematoma, pseudoaneurysm (especially with femoral artery cannulation), infection, accidental dislodgement of catheter leading to exsanguinations of blood, and accidental intra-arterial administration of vasoactive drugs. If an area appears ischemic, the catheter should be removed as soon as possible.
- Accidental drug injection may cause severe, irreversible damage to the hand.

SPECIAL CONSIDERATIONS

- The use of ultrasonographic guidance during arterial line placement has been demonstrated to significantly decrease the failure rate, complication rate, and number of attempts required for successful access.[2]
- Perform the Allen test to determine the patency of collateral blood flow and the contribution of the radial and ulnar arteries to the total blood flow of the hand. If ulnar perfusion is poor and a cannula occludes the radial artery, blood flow to the hand may be reduced.
  - The Allen test is performed by asking the patient to clench his or her hand. The ulnar and radial arteries are occluded with digital pressure.
  - The hand is unclenched and pressure over the ulnar artery is released. If there is good collateral perfusion, the palm should flush in less than 6 seconds.
  - The ability of Allen testing to predict complications is questionable. Practitioners must consider all factors. Longer direct compression on a punctured vessel should be applied after unsuccessful attempts in **coagulopathic** patients to prevent hematoma.
  - Lidocaine infiltration subcutaneously has been shown to reduce arterial vasospasm and should be considered prior to all cannulation attempts.

- If a difference in the measured pressure exists between two upper extremities, then the side with the higher pressure should be chosen as the cannulation site.

SUPPLIES

- Sterile gloves
- Betadine or chlorhexidine skin prep
- Bendable soft wrist board towel roll to extend the wrist joint
- Transparent sterile occlusive dressing (Tegaderm or Opsite)
- Arterial line kit (20-gauge catheter with 22-gauge introducer needle and guidewire); note differing kits for axillary and femoral cannulation
- Arterial line monitoring kit with 0.9% normal saline 500 mL in a pressurized bag
- Arterial line monitoring cable
- Suture material for femoral arterial insertion; 2.0 Silk suture
- Local anesthetic—lidocaine 1% or 2%

PROCEDURAL INSTRUCTIONS: PLACEMENT OF ARTERIAL CATHETER

- Gather all necessary equipment and bring to the bedside.
- Connect transducer to the pressurized normal saline bag and the monitoring cable
- Patient preparation
  - Explain risk and benefit of the procedure. Obtain procedural consent.
  - Identify patient with two identifiers (name, date of birth, medical record number, etc.).
  - Perform time out and mark the identified site of cannulation.
  - Perform Allen test for radial artery cannulation (see **FIGURE 17-1**).
    - Form a tight fist or raise the arm above the level of the heart.

FIGURE 17-1: Perform Allen test

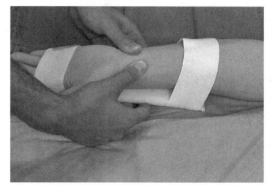

- Occlude both radial and ulnar arteries by applying direct pressure.
- Release the pressure on the ulnar artery and observe for presence of erythematous blush or pallor on the palmar surface of the hand.
- Presence of erythematous blush signifies patency of ulnar artery (positive Allen test) and pallor after 6 seconds indicates compromised ulnar artery.

PROCEDURE[3]

- Dorsiflex wrist and place over towel roll or bendable wrist board. Tape the forearm and wrist to the arm board or bedside table to allow for maximum exposure and access to the artery.
- Prep the cannulation site with povidone or chlorhexidine.
- Sterile drape at the entry site.
- Palpate pulsatile radial artery distally or 1–2 cm from the wrist joint. Infiltrate site of cannulation with lidocaine 1%.
- Use one of the following three methods.

Seldinger Technique

- Insert the arterial catheter at an angle of 30–60° (see **FIGURE 17-2**).
- A flash of bright, red-colored blood will be seen entering the column and will continue to rise.

FIGURE 17-2: Insert needle at 45° angle

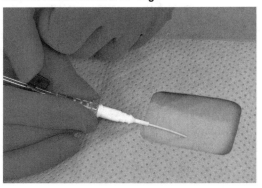

FIGURE 17-4: Remove wire

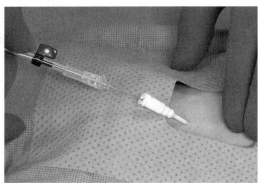

FIGURE 17-3: Advance wire through catheter

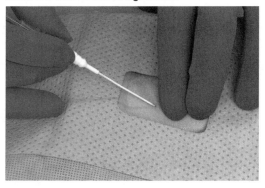

FIGURE 17-5: Attach catheter to pressure line

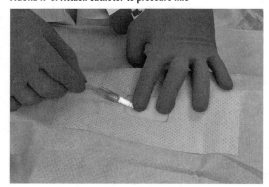

- Advance the guidewire, and using **Seldinger technique**, advance the catheter over the guidewire with a twisting motion (see **FIGURE 17-3**).

Transfixation Technique

- After obtaining flashback, advance the cannula a few millimeters, passing through the posterior wall of the artery.
- Remove the needle and withdraw the cannula until free pulsatile flow of blood is seen (see **FIGURE 17-4**).
- Pass a guidewire through the cannula and advance the cannula over the guidewire.

Direct Cannulation

- This technique is similar to venous cannulation.
- Following palpation and localization of the artery, advance the needle at a 30° angle.
- When free flow of blood is noted at the hub, the catheter is advanced over the needle.
- Connect the catheter to the pressurized arterial line tubing and observe for pressure waveform (see **FIGURE 17-5**).
- Secure the connections tightly, and apply transparent sterile dressing. Suture the catheter to the skin for femoral artery cannulation.
- Zero the arterial line monitoring system.

CATHETER REMOVAL

- Disconnect the arterial monitoring cable and then remove the transparent occlusive dressing.
- Apply a 4- × 4-inch gauze pad over the catheter entry site and remove the catheter while applying pressure.
- Hold pressure 5–10 minutes.
- Inspect the catheter for integrity.

AFTERCARE INSTRUCTIONS

- Inspect puncture site for the presence or development of a hematoma.
- Look for signs of arterial insufficiency on the digits of the hands (cyanosis, pallor, swelling) and signs of infection (discharge, erythema, swelling).
- Avoid strenuous activity for the next 24 hours on the extremity where the arterial line was placed.

► REFERENCES

1. Scheer B, Perel A, Pfeiffer UJ. Clinical review: complications and risk factors of peripheral arterial catheters used for haemodynamic monitoring in anaesthesia and intensive care medicine. *Crit Care*. 2002;6(3):199–204.
2. Shiver S, Blaivas M, Lyon M. A prospective comparison of ultrasound-guided and blindly placed radial arterial catheters. *Acad Emerg Med*. 2006;13(12):1275–1279.
3. Milzma D, Janchar T. Arterial puncture and cannulation. In: Roberts JR, Hedges JR, eds. *Clinical Procedures in Emergency Medicine*. 4th ed. Philadelphia, PA: W.B. Saunders; 2004:384–400.

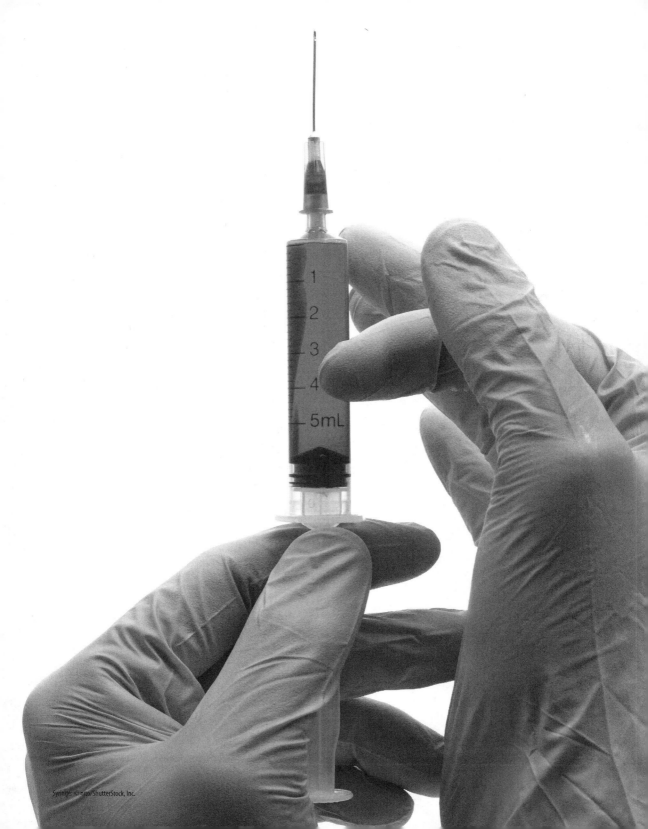

CHAPTER 18
Central Venous Line Insertion

Lisa A. Johnson, DrNP, CRNP, ACNP-BC

GOALS

▶ Monitor the central venous pressure in acutely ill patients to quantify fluid balance.

▶ Administer long-term pain medications, vasopressors, antibiotics, chemotherapy, and parenteral nutrition.

▶ Venous blood sampling.

OBJECTIVES

1. Discuss the rationale for central venous line placement.
2. Explain evidence-based indications for central venous line placement.
3. Describe contraindications associated with central venous line placement.
4. Describe the process for central venous line insertion.
5. Differentiate between proper and improper central venous line placement techniques.
6. Illustrate potential complications of central venous line insertion.

RATIONALE FOR PROCEDURE

- Indicated when other peripheral sites are unavailable or inaccessible.
- A central venous catheter (CVC) is needed for the infusion of **vasopressors** and hyperalimentation fluids.
- Central venous access is needed for placement of a pulmonary artery catheter or pacemaker, for performance of hemodialysis or plasmapheresis.

EVIDENCE-BASED INDICATIONS

- CVCs allow for the administration of intravenous fluids and critical medications such as antibiotics, hemodynamic support, certain chemotherapeutic agents, and total parenteral nutrition (TPN).
- Central venous lines allow for the measurement of central venous pressure (CVP).
- They can also be used during hemodialysis and plasmapheresis.

CONTRAINDICATIONS

- General contraindications for placement of a central venous line include thrombosis and infection at the site of the target vessel.
- Patients who have a pneumothorax or hemothorax on the contralateral side should not receive a central venous line.
- Uncooperative patients unable to undergo sedation and who have distortion of the anatomic landmarks from any cause should not receive a central venous line.
- Although coagulopathy is not a contraindication to central venous line insertion, extreme caution should be given to those with coagulopathies or on active anticoagulation therapy.
- Platelet transfusion should occur prior to the procedure to achieve a goal platelet count of at least 50,000.

- Other relative contraindications include patients receiving positive end-expiratory pressure (PEEP) mechanical ventilation and those with only one functioning lung.
- Keep in mind, no absolute contraindications are given as individual patient needs and risk/benefit must be weighed in the critical care setting.

COMPLICATIONS

- Immediate concerns of central venous line insertion include venous air embolism, pneumothorax, and **arterial puncture**.
- When the tip of the venous catheter is advanced into the thorax, negative intrathoracic pressures created during breathing can move air into the venous circulation through an open catheter and produce an **air embolism**.[1] In order to decrease the risk of embolism, the venous pressure needs to remain higher than the atmospheric pressure. Placing the patient in Trendelenburg position with the head of the bed 15° below the horizontal plane will decrease the risk of the procedure-related embolism.
- Clinicians should suspect an air embolism if the patient develops an acute onset of dyspnea during central venous line insertion. If a venous embolism is suspected, attach a syringe to the hub of the catheter immediately and aspirate air through the indwelling catheter. Also, place patients in the left lateral position in an effort to keep air in the right side of the heart. Despite these efforts, mortality is high in severe cases of venous air embolism.[1]
- Pneumothorax occurs in 1–6% of all CVC insertions. The higher incidence occurs with increased needle passes, emergency situations, and large catheter placement (those used for hemodialysis).[2]
- Other potential immediate complications include the induction of arrhythmias during the procedure. The majority of arrhythmias include ventricular ectopy; however, in 1%

of cases therapeutic intervention and catheter removal are necessary.[2] In addition, arterial puncture can occur. If an arterial puncture occurs, stop the procedure and place pressure on the site for 10 minutes.

- Infection is the main complication of indwelling catheters. The risk of infection is highest in the femoral vein insertion sites. Measures to decrease the risk of infection include choosing the appropriate insertion area, the use of proper hand hygiene, strict sterile technique during insertion and dressing changes, use of chlorhexidine, and the removal of the CVC as soon as possible. The Institute for Healthcare Improvement (IHI) recommends hospitals use a catheter line bundle to decrease the risk of central venous access bloodstream infections.

SPECIAL CONSIDERATIONS

- The use of **ultrasonographic guidance** during central venous line placement has been demonstrated to significantly decrease the failure rate, complication rate, and number of attempts required for successful access.

SUPPLIES

- Central line insertion kit—example shown in **FIGURE 18-1** (*Note*: It is important to become familiar with the central line insertion kit that your institution uses. While they are basically the same, there are minor differences among manufacturers. Most kits have a comprehensive list of inclusions on the package's outer wrap.)
- Rolled-up bath towel
- Paper tape measure
- Sterile saline flushes
- Skin preparation equipment
- Sterile gloves
- Sterile gown
- Face mask with splash guard
- Sterile drapes (sometimes included in kit)

FIGURE 18-1: Contents of central line kit

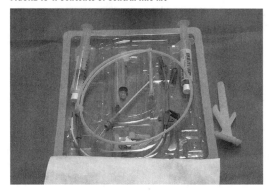

- Suture (sometimes included in kit)
- Lidocaine (sometimes included in kit)

PROCEDURAL INSTRUCTIONS

Vessel Selection and Anatomy

- Three primary veins are used for central line cannulation: the internal jugular, the subclavian, and the femoral vein. Most right-handed practitioners prefer to use the vessels on the right side of the patient's body. This will align the practitioner so the line can be inserted without the practitioner's dominant hand having to cross over.
- The internal jugular vein is the first choice of many practitioners. The internal jugular vein leads directly into the subclavian vein.
- When placing the central line, the patient should be positioned with his or her head turned to the contralateral side. In this position, the two heads of the sternocleidomastoid muscle and the clavicle create a triangle. The internal jugular vein sits in the vertex of the triangle between two heads of muscle. The carotid artery is located medial to the internal jugular vein. Information provided is directed to cannulating this vessel. It is important that the practitioner locates the carotid artery to avoid inadvertent cannulation.
- The subclavian vein is a continuation of the axillary vein. It is located beneath the clavicle

and just lateral to the subclavian artery. Veni-puncture should occur 1 cm lateral to the cur-vature of the middle third of the clavicle with the needle pointing horizontally directed at the sternal notch. At this point, the subclavian artery lies superior and posterior to the vein.

- The final site to consider is the femoral vein. The femoral vein can be located by palpat-ing the femoral artery pulse just below the inguinal crease. The vein should be can-nulated approximately 1 to 2 centimeters medial to the palpated pulse.
- It is important to note that ultrasound tech-nology is becoming an important tool in central line insertion; its use can definitively map the vessel and visualize the needle as it violates the vessel. If your institution has the capability for ultrasound, it is important to familiarize yourself with this technology.

Preparation and Positioning

- As with all invasive procedures, the process should be explained to the patient, the pa-tient's questions should be answered, and informed consent should be obtained. Seda-tion can also be considered. In the following example, preparation and placement infor-mation for a subclavian line will be provided.
- Catheter length is determined by measuring the patient's size. The catheter should termi-nate about 2 to 3 cm below the manubrios-ternal junction, in the superior vena cava, just above the right atrium. This distance can be measured with a tape measure.
- Prior to initiating the procedure for subclavian line placement, the patient must be optimally positioned. Ideally, the patient should be placed in Trendelenburg position to engorge the vessels and aid in visualization. An angle of 15° below the horizontal plane is ideal.
- Place a rolled towel or sheet between the shoulder blades to make the clavicles more prominent; this will help in identifying the anatomy. The patient's head should be turned to the contralateral side.

FIGURE 18-2: Cleanse insertion site area

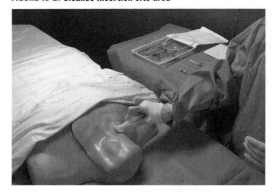

- It is important to find your landmarks for the chosen vessel before the area is prepped. Once the patient is sterile and draped, find-ing landmarks can be more difficult.
- Wash hands and put on gloves.
- Cleanse insertion site with chlorhexidine or another antiseptic cleanser as per your in-stitution's policy (see **FIGURE 18-2**). Prep an area that is larger than needed. For an internal jugular or subclavian site, prep from neck to nipple to axilla. The chlorhexidine needs a full 2 minutes to dry for the antimicrobial action to be fully effective.
- Remove gloves.

Setup and Insertion

- Ensure that all supplies needed are at the bedside. At this point, the practitioner should don sterile attire then drape the pa-tient in the standard sterile fashion. A fenes-trated drape is often included in the central line kit.
- Next, anesthetize the skin with lidocaine. Needle should be aimed at the ipsilateral nipple. Lidocaine injection should be sub-dermal, creating a wheal just beneath the skin. Continue to anesthetize the surround-ing area.
- Confirm your landmarks, and using a finder needle and gentle negative pressure, insert the needle bevel up until a flash of blood is

FIGURE 18-3: Insertion with needle bevel up

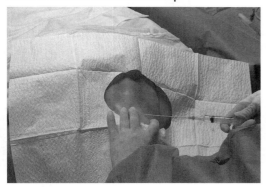

FIGURE 18-5: Guidewire placement

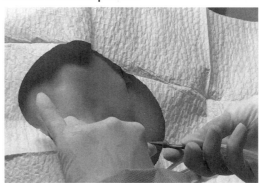

FIGURE 18-4: Aspirate until flashback visible

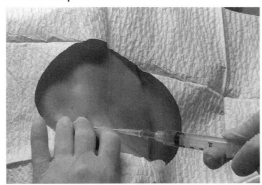

seen (see **FIGURE 18-3**). Note angle and depth of finder needle, and then remove. The goal of using a finder needle first is to find the vessel in a less traumatic manner.

- Using a larger needle (typically 18 gauge), follow the path of the finder needle using the same procedure. Apply gentle constant negative pressure until blood is seen in the syringe (see **FIGURE 18-4**). At this point, it may be necessary to determine if this is venous or arterial blood. Some central line insertion kits have a transducer tube that can be connected to the needle. This will help differentiate venous from arterial cannulation.

- Once a venous cannulation is determined, gently unscrew the syringe and remove, leaving the needle in place. Place your thumb over the exposed needle hub to help prevent an air embolism, then gently place the guidewire through the needle (see **FIGURE 18-5**). The wire should always move freely and easily. It is extremely important to hold the guidewire the entire time that it is in the body. At no time should the practitioner let go of the wire, because this may result in the wire inadvertently being pulled into the vein. Depending on the length of the guidewire, it should be inserted with approximately 10 cm left outside the body.

- Keeping a firm hold on the wire, remove the needle, sliding it out on top of the guidewire. Using the scalpel, make a small cut adjacent to the wire (see **FIGURE 18-6**). The blade should always face away from the wire to prevent inadvertently cutting the wire. Thread the dilator over the guidewire into the chest using gentle pressure. It is important to hold the guidewire during this portion. The dilator can then be removed.

- Flush the catheter. This can be done with the help of an assistant, or if the saline syringes are sterile, they can be placed directly on the field and the cap can be

FIGURE 18-6: **Use scalpel and hold wire**

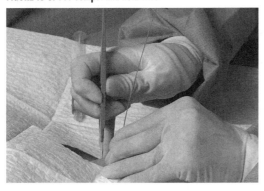

FIGURE 18-8: **Slide dark blue on guidewire**

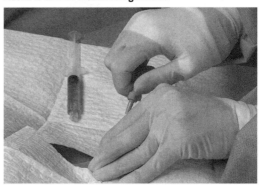

FIGURE 18-7: **Slide on guidewire**

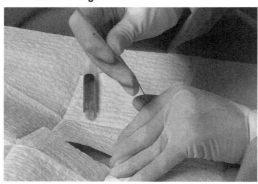

removed from the most distal lumen of the line, as this is where the wire will emerge. Most often, this is the brown port. The line is placed over the wire (see **FIGURE 18-7**).

Remove the wire once the catheter is in place (see **FIGURE 18-8**). Ensure that there is a blood return from all three lumens. Flush the lines and suture it in place.

- Post-insertion chest x-rays are needed to confirm placement of the central venous line. Optimally, a portable chest x-ray should be obtained with the patient in the upright position during exhalation (although often not possible in the critically ill population). The catheter tip should lie in the lower superior vena cava. The chest x-ray will determine proper placement and assess for pneumothorax. The CVC should not be used until confirmation of placement is attained by chest x-ray.

► REFERENCES

1. Marino PL. *The ICU Book*. 3rd ed. Philadelphia, PA: Lippincott, Williams & Wilkins; 2007.

2. Kusminsky RE. Complications of central venous catheters. *J Am Coll Surg*. 2007; 204(4):681–696.

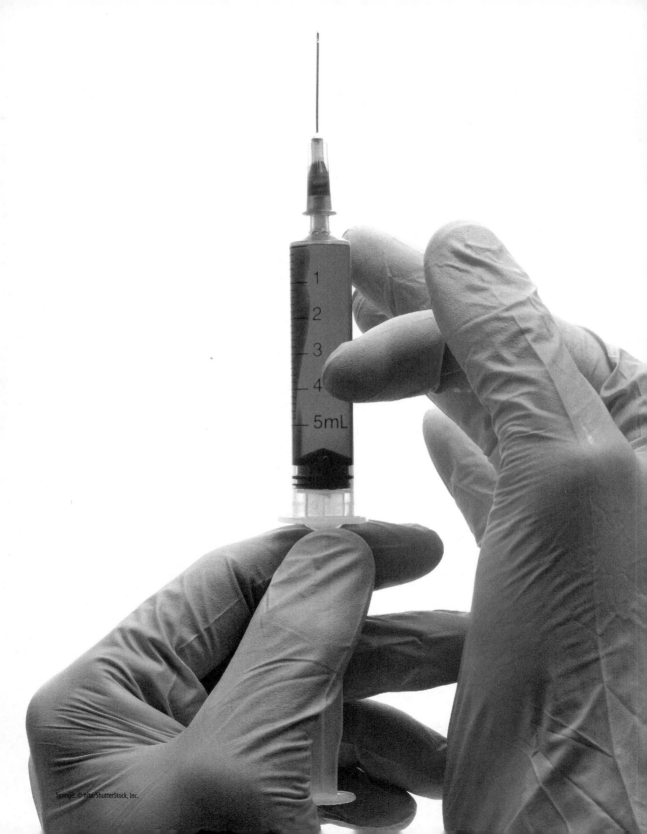

CHAPTER 19

Lumbar Puncture

Maha Lund, DHSc, PA-C
Nancy Hurwitz, PA-C, MHP

GOALS

► Reduce cerebrospinal fluid (CSF) pressure.

► Diagnose infectious central nervous system conditions and subarachnoid hemorrhage using CSF sampling.

► Increase intracranial pressure.

OBJECTIVES

1. List the indications for lumbar puncture.
2. List the contraindications for lumbar puncture.
3. Describe when a computed tomography (CT) scan is and is not required prior to lumbar puncture.
4. List and discuss the complications of lumbar puncture.
5. Describe the equipment employed for lumbar puncture.
6. Demonstrate a safe method for performing a lumbar puncture.

RATIONALE FOR PROCEDURE

- Diagnosis of central nervous system (CNS) infection
- Diagnosis of subarachnoid hemorrhage
- Infusion of anesthetic, chemotherapy, or contrast agents into the spinal canal
- Treatment of idiopathic intracranial hypertension
- Evaluation and diagnosis of demyelinating or inflammatory CNS processes

EVIDENCE-BASED INDICATIONS

- Suspected CNS infection (bacteria, *Cryptococcus*, virus, encephalitis, syphilis, Lyme disease)
- Suspected noninfectious meningitis (sarcoid, chemical, lupus)
- Suspected subarachnoid hemorrhage
- Diagnosis/staging/treatment of neoplastic disease
- Therapeutic reduction of CSF pressure
- Sampling of CSF
- CNS malignancy
- Guillain-Barré syndrome
- Pseudotumor cerebri (idiopathic intracranial hypertension)
- Normal pressure hydrocephalus
- Vasculitis
- Multiple sclerosis
- Therapeutic delivery
  - Antibiotics
  - Anesthetics
  - Chemotherapy
  - **Cerebrospinal fluid** removal
  - Injection of contrast material

CONTRAINDICATIONS

- Advanced degenerative arthritis
- Past spinal surgery resulting in significant scarring
- Congenital defects
- Infection over/at the intended site:
  - Cellulitis
  - Osteomyelitis
- Bleeding diathesis
- Cardiopulmonary instability
- Known or suspected increased intracranial pressure
- Uncorrected coagulopathy
- Skin infection near site
- Spinal cord trauma

COMPLICATIONS

In order of frequency:

- Post-spinal headache
- Infection:
  - At the site
  - Meningitis
- Hemorrhage or bleeding
- Minor neurologic symptoms: radicular pain or numbness
- Cerebral herniation
- Anaphylaxis
- Hearing impairment
- Sixth nerve palsy
- Formation of epidermoid tumor

SPECIAL CONSIDERATIONS

Pre-lumbar puncture CT is required if:

- Risk or suspicion of increased intracranial pressure
- Altered mental status
- Focal neurologic signs/symptoms
- Papilledema
- Focal seizure or unexplained seizure within 1 week of the **lumbar puncture**
- Risk for brain abscess
- Impaired cellular immunity

SUPPLIES

- Test tubes (3–4)
  - Three to four test tubes are provided for the collection of CSF (see **FIGURE 19-1**).

FIGURE 19-1: Test tubes

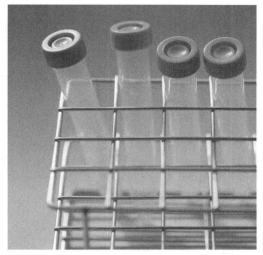

© Ann Cutting/Alamy Stock Photo

- ■ These should be opened and placed upright with tray setup.
- Manometer and tubing
  - ■ The manometer is used to measure the opening pressure of the CSF (see **FIGURE 19-2**). It is made of plastic tubes that connect together. The height of the CSF column can be read from the side of the manometer. It attaches to the top portion of the stopcock by the flexible manometer tubing.

- Three-way stopcock (see **FIGURE 19-3**)
  - ■ The stopcock connects the lumbar puncture needle to the manometer (or manometer tubing). It has a lever that controls which of the three openings of the stopcock are open. One connects the lumbar puncture needle to the stopcock and the stopcock to the manometer to measure opening pressures.
- Sterile sponges or sticks for application of Betadine
- Anesthetic vial for local anesthesia
  - ■ The lumbar puncture set is usually equipped with 1% lidocaine to use as a local anesthetic (see **FIGURE 19-4**).
- Band-Aid
  - ■ The adhesive bandage is placed over the lumbar puncture site at the completion of the procedure to prevent mild bleeding from the skin puncture site.
- Needles (see **FIGURE 19-5**)
- Fenestrated and non-fenestrated drape
- Povidone-iodine and tray
- Mask
- Sterile gloves
  - ■ Sterile gloves must be used for handling sterile equipment and in performing the lumbar puncture

FIGURE 19-2: Manometer

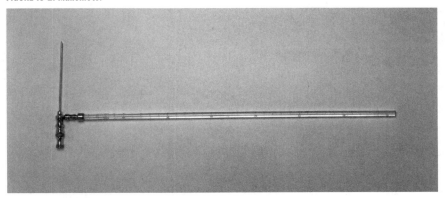

© Science & Society Picture Library/Getty Images

FIGURE 19-3: Stopcock

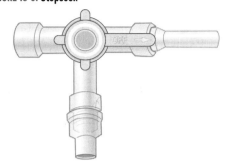

FIGURE 19-4: Lidocaine

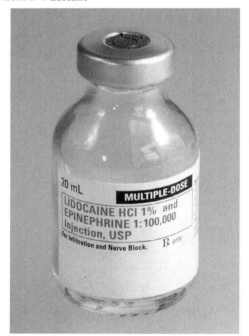

© Scott Camazine/Alamy Stock Photo

- Needles: two 22-gauge with **stylet** (typically 3.5-inch needle)
  - This needle has a removable stylet. The stylet should be in place anytime the lumbar puncture needle is advanced or removed. Quincke needles have a sharp cutting tip.
  - Traditional **Quincke needle** (beveled cutting tip)
    - Benefit: less expensive
- Needle alternatives:
  - **Sprotte needle** (with pencil point and side hole)
  - **Whitacre needle** (similar to Sprotte with smaller side hole)
    - Contraindicated for opening pressure and large-volume CSF drainage
  - Both considered to have lower risk of post-lumbar puncture headache
  - Both more expensive

FIGURE 19-5: Spinal needle

© saritwuttisan/iStockphoto

PROCEDURAL INSTRUCTIONS

- Informed consent
  - Patient or patient proxy must sign prior to procedure
- Positioning
  - Lateral knee-chest fetal position with neck, back, and limbs in flexion. Shoulders and hips perpendicular to the floor.
  - Alternative: Sitting with patient leaning forward over bedside table on two pillows. Indicated for obesity; significant lumbar degenerative joint disease; patients with respiratory compromise when lying flat; or spondylosis, rheumatoid arthritis, scoliosis, or ankylosing spondylitis.
  - Cannot measure opening pressure if patient in sitting position; result will be unreliable.
  - Once the patient is in the proper position, palpate the posterior superior iliac crests and imagine a line that connects the two. This line will cross the L3–L4 interspace. You may choose this space or one above or below to use in the adult patient. You may mark this space by pressing a plastic needle hub into the skin of patient's back at this space. The skin dent in this area will aid as a landmark.
  - Once the patient is properly positioned, prepare a stool for yourself and be sure that the bed is raised to a comfortable height to perform the procedure.
- Put on the mask and gown, open the lumbar puncture tray, and then put on the sterile gloves. It is essential to prepare all the equipment on the tray before proceeding.
- Place the collection tubes in their holders and remove their caps.
- Draw the local anesthetic into the provided syringe with the needle, and assemble the manometer.
- Apply the Betadine solution to the patient's back. Work in circular strokes starting at the skin dent placed on the patient's back and working concentrically outward. Using the same motion, wipe the excess off with sterile gauze.
- Next, pick up the blue sterile drape.
- Place the drape on the patient so the adhesive tape is oriented toward the patient and will stick to the area of their hips. Align the hole in the drape so that it exposes the area you intend to use for the lumbar puncture.
- Locate your chosen interspace (L3–L4 if using the posterior superior iliac crest line).
- Inject anesthesia: Local with 1% lidocaine subcutaneously with a 25- or 27-gauge needle, deeper with a 1.5-inch needle to anesthetize interspinous ligaments and muscles.
- Raise a skin bleb with the lidocaine. Proceed to anesthetize the deeper subcutaneous structures by directing the needle toward the umbilicus.
  - Bevel is turned in cephalad direction.
  - Layers the needle will penetrate:
    - Skin, superficial fascia, supraspinous ligament, interspinous ligament, ligamentum flavum, epidural space with fatty areolar tissue and internal vertebral plexus, dura, arachnoid membrane, subarachnoid space
- Following the skin puncture, advance the needle through the subcutaneous tissue and into the supraspinal and intraspinal ligaments. Advance the spinal needle, while continuing to ensure the needle is parallel to the bed and aimed at the umbilicus.
- Occasionally, while advancing the needle, resistance is encountered. If this should happen, withdraw the needle to the subcutaneous tissues and direct the needle slightly more cephalad. As the spinal needle is advanced deeper through the ligaments, repeatedly remove the stylet and check for CSF flow. In most instances as the needle is advanced, a "pop" may be noticed. This accompanies the piercing of the ligamentum flavum and dura mater. This often signifies that the needle is in the correct place. With sharp cutting needles, the provider may pass

through the ligamentum flavum and dura mater without feeling the pop.

- At this point, the stylet is removed and CSF should flow freely.
- When needle is in subarachnoid space and fluid returns, the manometer and 3-way stopcock are attached.
- If measuring opening pressure, the manometer is attached to the spinal needle and the stopcock opened to allow for CSF to fill the manometer.
- It is often helpful to have an assistant steady the top portion of the manometer, so the provider is free to manipulate the stopcock. The opening pressure is the pressure in the column after the fluid ceases to rise.
- Following the opening pressure measurement, the stopcock is turned so that the CSF drains out through the spigot and is collected into 1 of the 4 test tubes provided in the lumbar puncture kit.
- Opening pressure
  - Normal: 50–200 mmHg
  - Best measured with patient in lateral position with knees and hips slightly extended out of fetal position
  - Cannot be measured with patient in sitting position due to interference of hydrostatic pressure of the CSF column above the entry point
  - After pressure is measured, drain fluid from manometer into tube and allow additional fluid to drain
- If you are not measuring opening pressure, collect the CSF in the sequentially labeled test tubes (i.e., tube #1 gets CSF first, tube #4 gets CSF last). You need to collect approximately 3–5 mL of CSF per test tube.
- When the necessary CSF has been collected, the stylet is replaced into the spinal needle and the needle is withdrawn in one motion. Clean your patient's back and place a bandage over the puncture site.
- Fluid collection
  - Typical collection is 15–20 mL or 5 mL per tube. Up to 35 mL may be safely removed.

- Tube 1: protein, glucose, electrophoresis, and cell count
- Tube 2: culture, Gram stain, and cytology
- Tube 3: cell count and serology
- Tube 4: polymerase chain reaction and special testing
- Cell count is used in tubes 1 and 3 to differentiate traumatic tap (count should decrease) versus subarachnoid hemorrhage (no change in cell count).

POST PROCEDURE: POSITIONING

- Patient remains supine and flat for 30 minutes to 3 hours depending on practitioner preference. Studies have not proven there is any benefit to post-procedure rest.

POST PROCEDURE: RISKS AND COMPLICATIONS

Post-Lumbar Puncture Headaches

- There is a 1–70% risk of occurrence; studies vary widely. Possible mechanism: excessive leakage of CSF into paraspinous spaces leading to intracranial hypotension with stretching and expansion of pain-sensitive intracerebral veins. If the patient experiences a headache after the lumbar puncture, it is typically a frontal or occipital headache. Headaches may develop within 1–3 days after the procedure and typically last 3–5 days, although in rare occasions can last for up to 10 days.
  - Associated symptoms: nausea, vomiting, dizziness, tinnitus, and vision changes
  - Treatment: rest, hydration, analgesics, antiemetics, or blood patch

Hemorrhage

- Spinal subarachnoid hemorrhage: very rare
  - Leads to blockage of CSF outflow with resulting back and radicular pain, sphincter disturbances, and—very rarely—paraparesis

- Spinal subdural hematoma: very rare
- Requires surgical intervention and carries significant morbidity

Infection

- Local or meningitis: Rare and can be prevented with aseptic technique

Hearing Impairment: Rare

- It has been suggested that the mechanism of transient hearing loss after spinal anesthesia relates to aberrancy in the anatomy of the cochlear aqueduct, leading to increased flow of CSF through the cochlear aqueduct, which occurs in approximately 2 in 1000 patients. The increased flow in the aqueduct decreases the perilymphatic pressure when the CSF pressure decreases after a dural puncture. This decrease in perilymphatic pressure leads to an increase in the endolymphatic pressure, resulting in the formation of an endolymphatic hydrops. An endolymphatic hydrops displaces the hair cells on the basement membrane and results in low-frequency hearing loss.

Sixth Nerve Palsy (Abducens Palsy): Very Rare

- Transient with most patients recovering within days to weeks. Thought to be caused by nerve traction following CSF removal or intracranial hypotension.

Minor Neurologic Symptom

- Radicular pain or numbness
  - Caused by local nerve irritation from needle or instilled chemical during procedure
  - Typically transient

Cerebral Herniation

- Associated with underlying process causing increased intracranial pressure missed on original diagnostic plan. Should always be considered as a risk.

Anaphylaxis

- Could be caused by instilled chemical or by local anesthetic

Formation of Epidermoid Tumor: Rare

- May only become evident years after procedure
- Most likely in children ages 5–12 years who had lumbar puncture in infancy, but has also been reported in adults
- Could be caused by epidermoid tissue that is transplanted into the spinal canal during the lumbar puncture
- Suggested that this occurs when no stylet or a loosely fitting stylet is used and could be avoided by using a tightly fitting stylet

PEDIATRIC LUMBAR PUNCTURE

Indications

- Similar to that of adults including CSF infection, subarachnoid hemorrhage, pseudotumor cerebri, installation of chemotherapeutics or radiologic contrast, and removal of CSF

Contraindications

- Risk of increased intracranial pressure

Special Considerations

- Special consideration should be given to children with bleeding diathesis, cardiopulmonary instability, spina bifida, behavioral issues

Preparation

- Age-appropriate education for the patient should occur prior to the procedure.
- Consider EMLA cream (lidocaine 2.5% and prilocaine 2.5%) 30–60 minutes prior to procedure for superficial anesthesia.

- Consider procedural sedation if behavioral issues that will compromise the safety of the patient.
- Obtain signed consent from the parent or legal guardian.

Supplies

- 22-gauge stylet needle of appropriate length (1.5–3.5 inches depending on age and size of child)
- No manometer typically available in pediatric lumbar puncture kit
- Resuscitation equipment should be readily available

Procedure

The pediatric procedure varies from the adult lumbar puncture in the following ways:

- Typically no opening pressure is performed unless pseudotumor cerebri is the suspected diagnosis.
- Consider doing procedure under fluoroscopy if necessary (if structural abnormality, e.g., spina bifida).
- The stability of proper positioning is critical for the success of a pediatric lumbar puncture. Patient has to be held in position.
- When infants are held in position, monitor airway and watch for respiratory compromise.
- Lumbar puncture is performed at the level of the cauda equina:
  - Children younger than 12 months: at L2/L3 to L5/S1
  - Children older than 12 months: at L3/L4 to L4/L5
- Though many practitioners believe no local injection of anesthesia is necessary, studies show that the lumbar puncture is much more likely to be successful and less likely to be traumatic if lidocaine is used.
- The use of oral sucrose applied to a pacifier may be helpful to diminish pain in infants up to 6 months of age.
- For appropriate needle angle, the tip of the needle is to be pointed toward the umbilicus.
  - Typically 45° perpendicular to the spinous ligaments in children younger than 12 months of age
  - Typically 30° perpendicular to the spinous ligaments in children older than 12 months of age
- The stylet may be removed just after entry through the skin or can be left in place until a "pop" is felt as the needle penetrates the dura and enters the subarachnoid space.
- As with adults, the stylet should be replaced before removal of the needle.
- There is no indication to have children lie flat post procedure, as spinal headaches post lumbar puncture are very rarely reported in children.

INTERPRETATION OF RESULTS

Opening Pressure

- 50–200 mm in most patients
- May be up to 250 mm in obese patients

CSF Interpretation

- Cell count should be performed within 60 minutes, because cell counts decrease with time as cells will settle or adhere to tube walls.

White Blood Cells (WBCs): Normal up to 5

- Lymphocytes rarely predominate in bacterial meningitis (see **TABLE 19-1**).

Red Blood Cells (RBCs): Normal up to 5

- Traumatic tap may be considered in setting of normal WBC count.
- General rule: Subtract 1 WBC for every 500–1500 RBCs if traumatic tap.
- Calculable rule: Predicted RBC = RBC in CSF × (peripheral WBC/peripheral RBC).

Protein

- Can be elevated in traumatic tap, subarachnoid hemorrhage, insulin-dependent diabetes mellitus (IDDM), noninsulin-dependent

TABLE 19-1: CSF Analysis

	White Blood Cells	Protein	Glucose
Bacterial	Increased (> 1000/microL; especially polymorphonuclear leukocytes)	Increased (> 250 mg/dL)	Decreased (< 45 mg/dL)
Aseptic viral, tuberculosis, fungal, neoplastic, parasitic, parameningeal, partially treated bacterial	Increased or normal (elevated lymphocytes)	Increased	Normal
Albuminocytologic, Guillain-Barré syndrome	Normal	Increased or significantly increased	Normal

diabetes mellitus (NIDDM), and in infectious and noninfectious meningitis

- May remain elevated for weeks to months after meningitis

Glucose

- Abnormally low in cases of bacterial meningitis, mycobacterial/mycoplasmal/fungal CSF infections, malignancies, CSF sarcoid, and subarachnoid hemorrhage
- Normal in viral CSF infections but may not hold true

Lactate

- May be elevated in bacterial meningitis but is no better at predicting this diagnosis than the blood-to-CSF glucose ratio and is not routinely used

Cytology

- May be useful in diagnosing malignancy but requires 10–15 mL of fluid

Immunoglobulins and Oligoclonal Bands

- May be elevated in any disorder that may disrupt the blood–brain barrier
  - For example: multiple sclerosis, neurologic Lyme disease, brain tumors, autoimmune disease, lymphoproliferative disease

Gram Stain

- Necessary to help identify original organism to guide treatment while awaiting culture results

Culture

- Used for definitive identification of causative organism
- Results will not be available until after 12–48 hours of growth
- Imperative in the long run, not helpful in the immediate treatment of the patient

▶ ADDITIONAL READING

Campbell WW. *DeJong's the Neurological Examination*. Philadelphia, PA: Lippincott Williams & Wilkins; 2005.

Wachter RM, Goldman L, Hollander H. *Hospital Medicine*. 2nd ed. Philadelphia, PA: Lippincott Williams & Wilkins; 2005.

Irwin RS, Rippe JM. *Irwin and Rippe's Intensive Care Medicine*. Philadelphia, PA: Lippincott Williams & Wilkins; 2011.

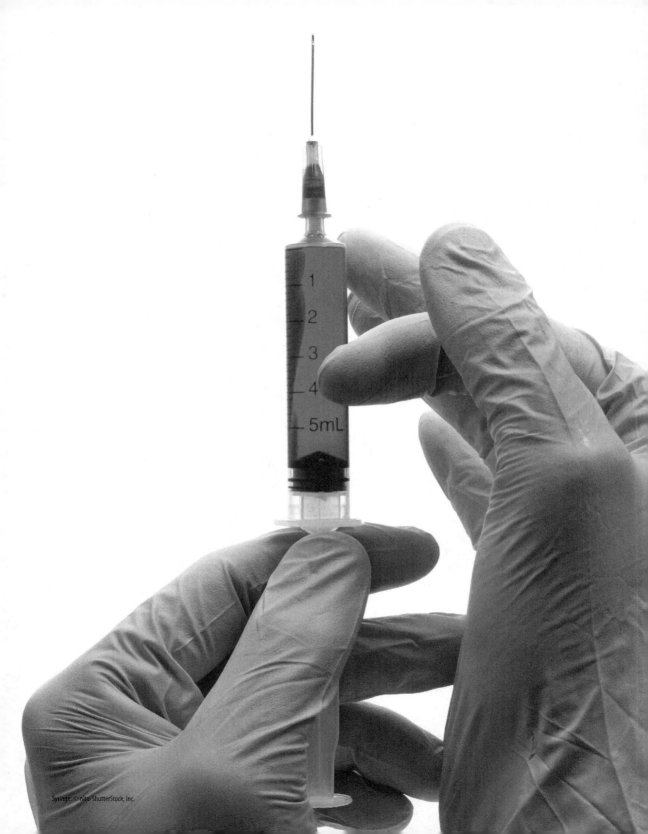

CHAPTER 20

Pulmonary Artery Catheterization (PAC) or Swan-Ganz Catheterization

Sharon Griswold-Theodorson, MD, MPH
James Connolly, MD
Jessica Parsons, MD

GOALS

▶ Understand the indications for performing pulmonary artery catheterization.

▶ Understand the effect of pulmonary artery catheterization on patient management.

OBJECTIVES

1. Describe the evidence-based recommendations for pulmonary artery catheterization (PAC).
2. Explain the risks and benefits of PAC.
3. Understand the possible complications from performing the procedure.

RATIONALE FOR PROCEDURE

- Unlike many procedures done for their singularity of purpose, PAC is unique in its use for treatment, diagnosis, and monitoring of the patient. Initially, PAC was performed in cardiac catheterization laboratories as an adjunct to decision making regarding cardiothoracic surgery.[1] The use of pulmonary artery (PA) catheters did not become commonplace until the 1970s, with the introduction of flow-directed, balloon-tipped catheters, now commonly called Swan-Ganz catheters (SGCs).[2] Originally conceived by Jeremy Swan as he watched sailboats from a Santa Monica beach, the idea he developed was to use an inflatable balloon to "sail" a catheter into the pulmonary artery via the right side of the heart.[3] For the following 2 decades, PA catheters provided enhanced understanding of cardiopulmonary pathophysiology through measures of cardiac output, systemic and pulmonary vascular resistance, and right and left heart-filling pressures.[4] The use of SGCs soon diffused from post-**myocardial infarction** management to the monitoring and care of other critically ill patients, as it was established that clinical evaluation of a patient's hemodynamic status based on clinical judgment by the bedside physician may be unreliable at best.[5] The belief at the time was that through PAC, individual pharmacotherapeutic interventions could be utilized, with real-time monitoring of patient response and data extraction. PACs could be used to gather crucial information, and together with clinical evaluation, allow clinicians to titrate fluids, **inotropes**, **vasopressors**, and **vasodilators** to optimize oxygen delivery to tissues.[6] However, throughout the history of medicine, interventions perceived initially as revolutionary often are not subjected to intense clinical and scientifically validated studies, which verify their usefulness as such. The effects of PAC on patient outcomes were not tested in randomized trials until after almost 40 years of use.

- In the 1980s, observational studies began to emerge questioning the safety and efficacy of the PA catheter, suggesting higher mortality rates for patients receiving PAC.[7,8] Subsequently, 5 large, randomized trials of PAC failed to demonstrate a significant clinical benefit to patients. These 5 trials are compelling, because they covered different study designs and patient populations, but arrived at similar results.[9-12] Given this confluence of data, the recent recommendations are against routine use of PAC in shock and do not recommend the PA catheter for any clinical scenario.[13] However, other meta-analyses have found select surgical populations in which the placement of a PA catheter has been beneficial[14] (see evidence-based indications later in this chapter).

- Data that can be collected and inferred when using a PA catheter include:[15]

  - Right heart pressures:
    - Right atrial pressure (RAP; see **FIGURE 20-1**)
    - Pulmonary artery pressures (see **FIGURE 20-2**)
      - Pulmonary artery systolic (PAS)
      - Pulmonary artery diastolic (PAD)
      - Pulmonary artery mean (PAM)
      - Pulmonary artery occlusion pressure (PAOP; see **FIGURE 20-3**)
- Mixed venous oxygen saturation (SvO_2) monitoring
- Intermittent measurement of right heart oxygen saturation to assess left–right shunt
- Continuous cardiac output (CCO)
- Right ventricular ejection fraction (RVEF; see **FIGURE 20-4**)
- Right ventricular end-diastolic volume (RVEDV) is continuous
- Systemic vascular resistance (SVR and SVRI)

EVIDENCE-BASED INDICATIONS

- The use of PA catheters remains controversial in the literature, with a multitude of studies in fact showing little to no benefit from PA catheter use, while others suggest

FIGURE 20-1: Normal insertion pressures and waveform tracings: right atrial/central venous pressure (RA/CVP)

Right Atrial/
Central Venous Pressure
(RA/CVP)

ECG

a c v   a c v   a c v   RA

2–6 mmHg
Mean 4 mmHg
a - atrial systole
c - backward bulging from tricuspid valve closure
v - atrial filling, ventricular systole

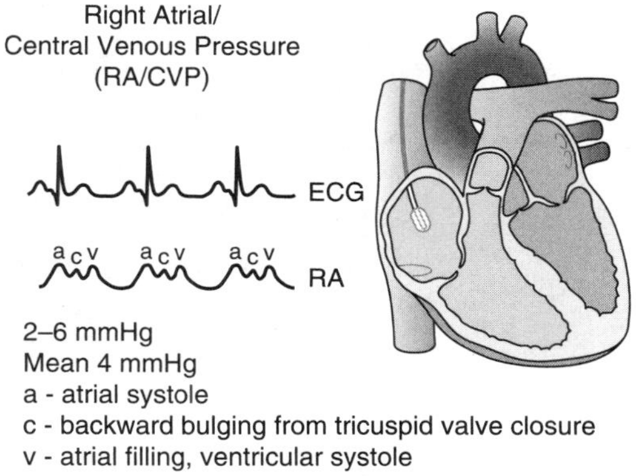

FIGURE 20-2: Normal insertion pressures and waveform tracings: pulmonary artery

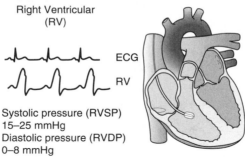

Right Ventricular
(RV)

ECG

RV

Systolic pressure (RVSP)
15–25 mmHg
Diastolic pressure (RVDP)
0–8 mmHg

FIGURE 20-3: Normal insertion pressures and waveform tracings: pulmonary artery occlusion pressure (PAOP)

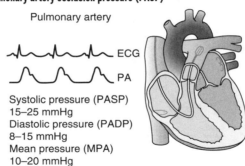

Pulmonary artery

ECG

PA

Systolic pressure (PASP)
15–25 mmHg
Diastolic pressure (PADP)
8–15 mmHg
Mean pressure (MPA)
10–20 mmHg

FIGURE 20-4: Normal insertion pressures and waveform tracings: right ventricular

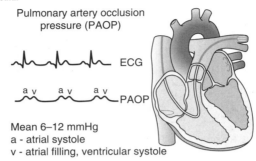

Pulmonary artery occlusion pressure (PAOP)

ECG

PAOP

Mean 6–12 mmHg
a - atrial systole
v - atrial filling, ventricular systole

increased mortality and morbidity. Cooper and colleagues performed an evidence-based review of the existing literature and constructed evidence-based recommendations for use of PA catheters, with several surprising results.[15] Strict evidence-based benefits from use of PA catheters have been demonstrated only in a few select scenarios, primarily in perioperative monitoring of high-risk surgical patients, hip fractures, or certain vascular limb surgeries. As noted previously, the evidence does not show a benefit to mixed intensive care unit (ICU) patients (level 1B).[15] (See **TABLE 20-1**.)

TABLE 20-1: Recommendation for PAC for Different Populations

Population	Recommendation	Level and Grade
Mixed ICU	Goal-oriented hemodynamic therapy does not improve patient outcome.	IB
Mixed ICU	PAC does not improve patient outcome.	IIV
High-risk surgical patients	Preoperative goal-oriented hemodynamic therapy improves patient outcome.	IIC
Hip fracture	Perioperative monitoring with PAC improves patient outcome.	IIC
Vascular surgery **Elective AAA** **Limb salvage**	Perioperative monitoring with PAC does not improve outcome. Preoperative hemodynamic intervention improves outcome.	IIC IIC
Coronary artery bypass surgery	PAC does not improve outcome, even in highest risk class.	IIID

TABLE 20-1: Recommendation for PAC for Different Populations (continued)

Mixed ICU, cardiac surgery	Oximetric catheters reduce neither laboratory costs nor cardiac output determinations.	IIC
Myocardial infarction	PAC does not worsen patient outcome in CHF.	IIID

AAA = abdominal aortic aneurysm; CHF = congestive heart failure; ICU = intensive care unit; PAC = pulmonary artery catheterization.

CONTRAINDICATIONS

Contraindications to placement of a PA catheter are similar to those of general central line placement. All contraindications are relative and should be considered in a broader overall picture of the patient and his or her condition.
- General
  - Extremes of weight
  - Vasculitis
  - Prior injection of sclerosing agents
  - Distorted local anatomy
  - Prior long-term venous cannulation
  - Bleeding disorders
  - Anticoagulation or thrombolytic therapy (relative)
  - Previous radiation therapy
  - Suspected vascular injury
  - Combative patients
  - Inexperienced, unsupervised operator
- Subclavian vein
  - Chest wall deformities
  - Chronic obstructive pulmonary disease (COPD)
  - Pneumothorax on the contralateral side
- Jugular vein
  - Intravenous drug abuse via the jugular veins

COMPLICATIONS[16]

- Carotid artery puncture or cannulation secondary to the proximity of the internal jugular (IJ)
- Pulmonary artery rupture possible due to balloon overinflation.

- Pneumothorax (air in pleural space collapsing the lung); IJ approach has a lower incidence of a pneumothorax than a subclavian or low anterior IJ approach.
- Patients with overinflated lungs (i.e., COPD or PEEP) may have an elevated risk of pneumothorax, especially with a subclavian approach.
- Hemothorax (blood in pleural space, collapsing the lung) secondary to artery puncture or laceration
- Hemorrhage within chest (hemothorax, tamponade) from artery injury or from insertion site
- Thoracic duct puncture or laceration
- Air embolism, increased risk in patients who are spontaneously breathing (negative pressure) as opposed to mechanical ventilation (positive pressure)
- *In situ* complications, vessel damage, hematoma, thrombosis, dysrhythmia, or cardiac perforation

SPECIAL CONSIDERATIONS

- Placing a Swan-Ganz or PA catheter can be a time-consuming process. It is important to be wary of this and arrange for proper support staff and monitoring of other patients while the operating physician and support team are occupied. The time from when the decision is made to place the line to the time that catheter-based treatments and interventions begin averages approximately 2 hours.[17]

- Patient position is essential for a successful outcome. Patient positioning should be similar to that of other central line placement. If IJ access is desired, the patient should be placed in a mild Trendelenburg position, which facilitates maximum engorgement of the IJ for easier needle cannulation. Further, the bed and patient should be positioned in such a position and height to allow the operator to easily palpate all relevant anatomy, while maintaining maximum comfort for both operator and patient.
- The operator may wish to consider a short-acting benzodiazepine (e.g., midazolam) for patients who are awake or exceedingly anxious.

SUPPLIES

- See **FIGURE 20-5**
- Three 2% chlorhexidine skin preps
- Sterile gloves and gown for each operator
- Face shield and cap for each operator and assistant
- 4- × 4-inch sterile gauze pads
- Sterile ultrasound probe cover and sterile ultrasound jelly
- 10 mL of 1% or 2% lidocaine, without epinephrine
- Sterile drape, preferably with precut adhesive opening for insertion site
- 25-gauge or similar needle with 3- to 10-mL lock-tip syringe
- 3.5-cm, 22-gauge needle with 5-mL slip-tip syringe

FIGURE 20-5: Prepare supplies

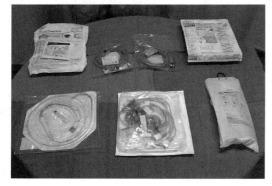

- 6-cm, 18-gauge large-bore needle with 5-mL slip-tip syringe
- J-tip guidewire
- 6-cm, 18-gauge transduction catheter
- Transduction tubing
- Soft-tissue dilator
- Three sterile saline line flushes
- Swan-Ganz catheter
- 2-0 or similar silk sutures on a straight needle, or other non-suture line-to-skin adhesion kit
- BioPatch
- Large Tegaderm

PROCEDURAL INSTRUCTIONS

- The first step is to choose the safest and most effective site for catheter placement after considering the risks and benefits of each location. The risks and benefits for each site—IJ versus subclavian versus brachial—are similar to central line placement and are discussed elsewhere. In general, however, the left subclavian or right IJ best facilitates placement of the catheter into the pulmonary artery. As a matter of general practice, femoral lines should be avoided secondary to concerns regarding increased rates of infection in this anatomic area.
- The most crucial component of the procedure for reducing infectious complications is the preparation of the procedural field. A wide field using sterile draping should be prepared with strict adherence to an aseptic technique. Prior to placement of the drape, a wide area surrounding the intended insertion site should be cleaned with 2% chlorhexidine. After placing the drape, the area should be cleaned 2 additional times, with adequate drying time between each application. Other components of aseptic technique, including hand washing and use of full barrier precautions, are covered elsewhere.
- After re-identifying anatomic structures via palpation, or preferably via ultrasound guidance, the insertion site should be infiltrated with a local anesthetic, typically 1% or 2%

lidocaine (without epinephrine), followed by superficial and deep structures along the anticipated needle tract. For subclavian approaches, the periosteum should also be anesthetized.

- An introducer needle should then be used to cannulate the previously identified vein. This is done in nearly identical fashion to insertion of other central venous catheters, typically utilizing the modified Seldinger technique. Once the wire has been successfully placed, the next step is to insert the pulmonary artery catheter over the wire and into the vessel, again, similar to other central line placement techniques. However, one key difference is that the PA catheter should be oriented so that its curve facilitates passage through the cardiac chambers. As the catheter is advanced through the introducer, the pressure at the tip should be transduced.

- The catheter balloon may be safely inflated once the pressure tracing indicates that the tip of the catheter is in the right atrium (see **FIGURE 20-6**). When inflating the balloon, if excessive resistance is met, it most likely indicates malpositioning of the catheter tip. Repositioning should be attempted before re-inflating the balloon.

- An important concept to keep in mind at all times is that after reaching the atrium with catheter tip, whenever the catheter is to be advanced, the balloon should be inflated (see **FIGURE 20-7**). Whenever it is to be withdrawn, the balloon should be deflated.

FIGURE 20-7: Insert catheter into sterile covering

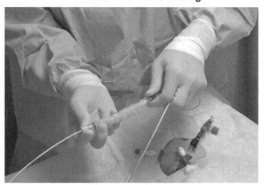

- Whenever the operator is attempting to advance the catheter, it is essential that he or she have an unobstructed view of the hemodynamic monitor (see **FIGURE 20-8**). Pressure tracings allow the operator to deduce the location of the catheter tip.

- The systolic pressure will increase significantly as the catheter tip crosses from the right atrium (RA) to the right ventricle (RV). This risk of arrhythmia is greatest while the catheter tip is in the RV; thus, the catheter should be advanced as quickly as possible from the RV to the PA. As the catheter passes into the PA, the diastolic pressure will increase and a characteristic dicrotic notch will appear in the waveform (see **FIGURE 20-9**). The catheter should continue to be slowly advanced until the pulmonary capillary wedge pressure (PCWP) is identified by a decrease in pressure,

FIGURE 20-6: Test catheter balloon

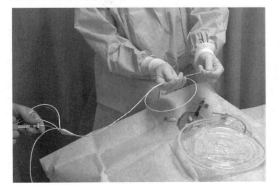

FIGURE 20-8: Advance catheter while monitoring pressure waves

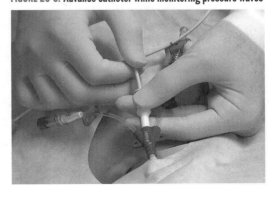

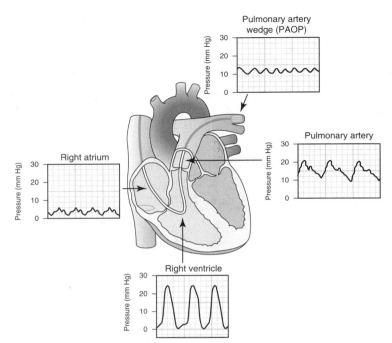

Pulmonary artery wedge (PAOP)

Pulmonary artery

Right atrium

Right ventricle

FIGURE 20-9: Tracings obtained in the right atrium or pulmonary capillary wedge position share similar morphology. The transition from the right ventricle to the pulmonary artery tracing can be identified by the increase in diastolic pressure and the presence of a dicrotic notch. The diastolic "step-up" results from the transducer crossing the pulmonic valve; the dicrotic notch reflects closing of the pulmonic valve

Reproduced from Marino PI. The ICU Book, Philadelphia, Lea and Febiger, 1991, p. 103.

combined with a change in waveform. The balloon should then be deflated and the PA tracing should reappear if placed correctly. If the PCWP tracing remains after deflating the balloon, or if the origin of the tracing is unclear, the catheter balloon should be withdrawn until a clear PA waveform emerges.

- If more than 30 cm of the catheter has been advanced, but no PA waveform has been obtained, it is likely that the catheter has coiled within the RV. If this occurs, deflate the balloon and withdraw the catheter until the RA waveform reappears. Another attempt can then be made at advancing the catheter.

- The catheter tip balloon has a maximum volume of 1.5 mL. A successful placement and final position of the catheter can be determined when a PCWP is obtained whenever 75–100% of the balloon is inflated (see **FIGURE 20-10**). If less than 1 mL is required to obtain a PCWP, the tip of the catheter is most likely in the distal PA and further insufflation could risk vessel rupture. In this situation the balloon should be deflated and withdrawn incrementally until proper placement

FIGURE 20-10: Lock catheter in place after assuring proper balloon placement

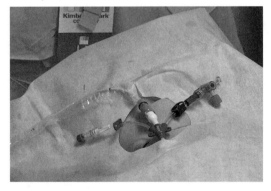

is found. On the other hand, if the balloon is fully inflated and fails to elicit a PCWP, or does so only after 2–3 seconds, the tip has likely not been advanced far enough. The catheter should thus be advanced incrementally until the desired waveform is obtained.

- Similar to any central line, a chest radiograph should be obtained to confirm the position of the catheter. Daily chest films may be desired to monitor for tip migration.

► REFERENCES

1. Dexter L, Haynes FW, Burwell CS, et al. Studies of congenital heart disease. I. Technique of venous catheterization as a diagnostic procedure 1. *J Clin Invest.* 1947;26(3):547–553.

2. Swan HJ, Ganz W, Forrester J, et al. Catheterization of the heart in man with use of a flow-directed balloon-tipped catheter. *N Engl J Med.* 1970;283(9):447–451.

3. Swan HJ. Pulmonary artery catheterization: development. In: Tobin MJ, ed. *Principles and Practice of Intensive Care Monitoring.* New York, NY: McGraw-Hill Health Professions Division; 1998.

4. Fowler RA, Cook DJ. The arc of the pulmonary artery catheter. *JAMA.* 2003;290(20):2732–2734.

5. Connors AF, Jr., Dawson NV, Shaw PK, et al. Hemodynamic status in critically ill patients with and without acute heart disease. *Chest.* 1990;98(5):1200–1206.

6. Rubenfeld GD, McNamara-Aslin E, Rubinson L. The pulmonary artery catheter, 1967–2007: rest in peace? *JAMA.* 2007;298:458–461.

7. Zion MM, Balkin J, Rosenmann D, et al. Use of pulmonary artery catheters in patients with acute myocardial infarction. Analysis of experience in 5,841 patients in the SPRINT Registry. SPRINT Study Group. *Chest.* 1990;98(6):1331–1335.

8. Gore JM, Goldberg RJ, Spodick DH, et al. A community-wide assessment of the use of pulmonary artery catheters in patients with acute myocardial infarction. *Chest.* 1987;92(4):721–727.

9. Binanay C, Califf RM, Hasselblad V, et al. Evaluation study of congestive heart failure and pulmonary artery catheterization effectiveness: the ESCAPE trial. *JAMA.* 2005;294:1625–1633.

10. Sandham JD, Hull RD, Brant RF, et al. A randomized, controlled trial of the use of pulmonary-artery catheters in high-risk surgical patients. *N Engl J Med.* 2003;348:5–14.

11. Richard C, Warszawski J, Anguel N, et al. Early use of the pulmonary artery catheter and outcomes in patients with shock and acute respiratory distress syndrome: a randomized controlled trial. *JAMA.* 2003;290:2713–2720.

12. Wheeler AP, Bernard GR, Thompson BT, et al. Pulmonary-artery versus central venous catheter to guide treatment of acute lung injury. *N Engl J Med.* 2006;354:2213–2224.

13. Antonelli M, Levy M, Andrews PJ, et al. Hemodynamic monitoring in shock and implications for management. International Consensus Conference, Paris, France, 27–28 April 2006. *Intensive Care Med.* 2007;33(4):575–590.

14. Wiener RS, Welch HG. Trends in the use of the pulmonary artery catheter in the United States, 1993–2004. *JAMA.* 2007;298:423–429. Sciences EL. Swan-Ganz Catheters.

15. Cooper AB, Doig GS, Sibbald WJ. Pulmonary artery catheters in the critically ill: an overview using the methodology of evidence-based medicine. *Critical Care Clinics.* 1996;12(4):777–794.

16. Boyd KD, Thomas SJ, Gold J, Boyd AD. A prospective study of complications of pulmonary artery catheterizations in 500 consecutive patients. *Chest.* Sep 1983;84(3):245–249.

17. Lefrant JY, Muller L, Bruelle P, et al. Insertion time of the pulmonary artery catheter in critically ill patients. *Crit Care Med.* Feb 2000;28(2):355–359.

► ADDITIONAL READING

Marino P. The pulmonary artery catheter. In: *The ICU Book.* 4th ed. Philadelphia, PA: Lippincott Williams & Wilkins; 2014: 135–150

McNeil C, Rezaie S, Adams B. Central venous catheterization and central venous pressure monitoring In: Roberts JR, ed., *Roberts and Hedges' Clinical Procedures in Emergency Medicine.* Philadelphia, PA: Elsevier; 2014: 397–431.

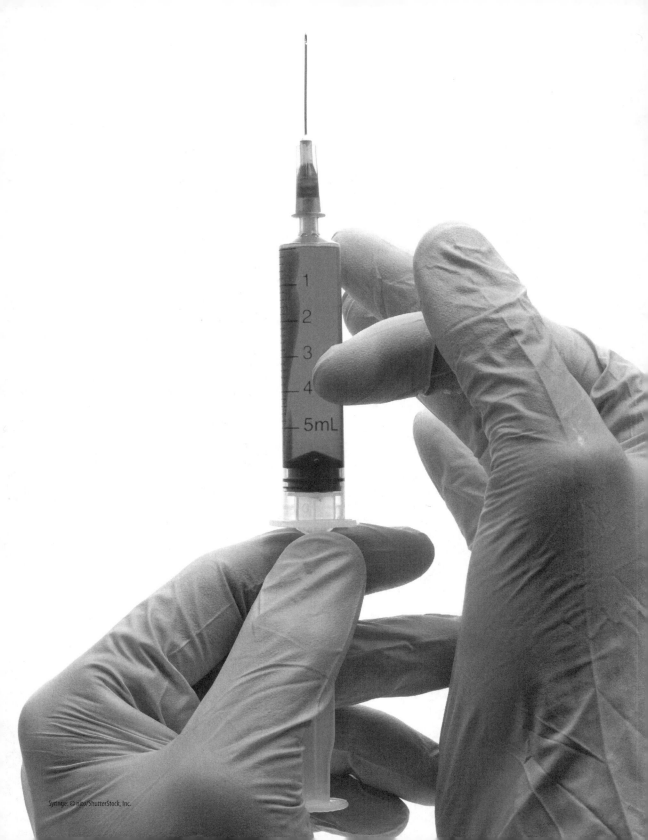

CHAPTER 21

Endotracheal Intubation

Lew Bennett, CRNA, DNP
Ferne M. Cohen, CRNA, MSN, EdD

GOAL

▶ Ensure airway patency in patients demonstrating respiratory insufficiency or those at risk for pulmonary aspiration.

OBJECTIVES

1. Describe the indications, contraindications, and rationale for performing endotracheal intubation.
2. Identify and describe common complications associated with endotracheal intubation.
3. Describe the essential anatomy and physiology associated with the performance of endotracheal intubation.
4. Identify the supplies and equipment needed for performing endotracheal intubation and their proper use.
5. Identify the important aspects of patient care following endotracheal intubation.

RATIONALE FOR PROCEDURE

- **Endotracheal intubation** is performed to improve oxygenation and ventilation and to protect the lungs from aspiration.

EVIDENCE-BASED INDICATIONS[1,2]

- Inadequate ventilation and oxygenation due to impaired cardiac, respiratory, or neurologic status
- Failure of conventional methods to maintain airway patency
- Impaired airway patency due to airway edema or upper airway obstruction
- Protection against aspiration

CONTRAINDICATIONS

- A provider who is unskilled in airway management
- Nasal intubation in patients with any type of bleeding disorder (including use of blood thinners), nasal deformity, facial/head trauma, or basal skull fracture

COMPLICATIONS[3]

- Undiagnosed esophageal intubation
- Lip laceration
- Dental damage
- Sore throat
- Corneal abrasion during laryngoscopy
- Bloody airway
- Inability to intubate
- Hypoxemia
- Damage to vocal cord(s)
- Vomiting and aspiration
- Right main stem intubation
- **Laryngospasm** prior to intubation
- Bronchospasm after intubation
- Aspiration pneumonia
- Failure to intubate leading to hypoxia and cardiac arrest

SPECIAL CONSIDERATIONS

- Evaluate the need for ventilatory support by assessing the patient's current respiratory, cardiac, and neurologic status.
- Auscultate all lung fields to assess if breath sounds are clear, equal, distant, or absent.[1]
- Perform a chin lift or jaw thrust if patient demonstrates signs and symptoms of upper airway obstruction (stridor, snoring).[4]
- An oral or nasal airway to move the tongue and **epiglottis** away from the posterior pharyngeal wall may alleviate airway obstruction.
  - An oral airway stimulates the gag reflex, promotes coughing or retching, and is not well tolerated by an awake patient.
  - A nasal airway is better tolerated in an awake patient but contraindicated if the patient is anticoagulated, has a bleeding tendency, or has a basilar skull fracture.[4]

ADVANTAGES

- Ability to oxygenate and ventilate a patient who is unable to maintain a patent airway

DISADVANTAGES

- Requires skill in airway management to perform task

SUPPLIES[5-9]

- Non-sterile gloves; if patient is latex allergic, ensure that gloves are latex-free
- Eye protection and face mask for the clinician
- Appropriately sized Macintosh blade (usually size 3 or 4) or Miller blade (usually size 2 or 3)
- Laryngoscope handle
- Endotracheal tube stylet
- Appropriately sized cuffed endotracheal tube (ETT); size is based upon patient age,

gender, and anatomic considerations (common adult ETT sizes 6.5, 7.0, 7.5, 8.0)

- 10-mL syringe used to inflate ETT cuff
- Appropriately sized oral airway and tongue blade
- Device to measure end-tidal carbon dioxide level (easy cap or end-tidal carbon dioxide [ETCO$_2$] monitor)
- Suction device with Yankauer and/or soft tip tracheal suction catheter
- Stethoscope to confirm breath sounds
- Adhesive tape to secure ETT
- Bag-valve mask (BVM) to provide positive pressure ventilation
- Medications to provide topical anesthesia, sedation, and paralysis
- Back-up equipment
  - **Supraglottic airway device** to provide positive pressure ventilation if intubation unsuccessful
  - Video laryngoscope[7]

PROCEDURAL INSTRUCTIONS[5-7]

- Explain procedure to patient in comprehensible language if awake and oriented.
- Perform **airway assessment** to determine potential for a difficult intubation; evaluate degree of mouth opening, quality of dentition, tongue size, neck circumference, and cervical mobility.[7]
- Assemble and test equipment prior to intubation.
- Ensure basic patient monitoring to include electrocardiogram (ECG), pulse oximeter, and blood pressure.
- Obtain intravenous access to administer sedatives or paralytics.
- Don protective eyewear, facemask, and gloves.
- Place patient into the **sniffing position** unless cervical-spine issues mandate neutral neck position.
- Deliver a 10-liter per minute flow of 100% oxygen via a BVM to **preoxygenate** the patient.
- If unable to ventilate, perform a chin lift if there are no contraindications.

- A jaw thrust can be used for challenging airways or uncleared cervical spine (**FIGURE 21-1**).
- For an awake patient, intravenous sedatives may include a combination of short-acting medications such as fentanyl, midazolam, or small incremental boluses of propofol (10–20 mg) titrated until the desired level of sedation is achieved.
- If the patient becomes apneic or a neuromuscular blocking agent is administered, administer positive pressure ventilation via a BVM.
- Effective ventilation requires a tight seal between the patient's face and BVM.

FIGURE 21-1: Jaw thrust

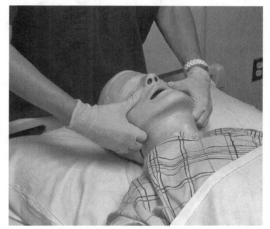

- Hold the mask tightly over the patient's mouth and nose with the thumb and index fingers of the left hand, with the 3rd–5th fingers being used to lift the chin. The right hand is used to squeeze the BVM (see **FIGURE 21-2**).
- For the two-handed ambu bag technique, see **FIGURE 21-3**.
- Hold the laryngoscope in the left hand.
- Open patient's mouth.
- Insert the laryngoscope blade into the right side of the mouth and sweep tongue left.
  - If using a Macintosh blade, advance the blade into the **vallecula** and lift epiglottis toward the patient's feet to expose vocal cords and glottis opening (examples of Macintosh blades are in **FIGURE 21-4**).

FIGURE 21-2: One-handed ambu bag technique

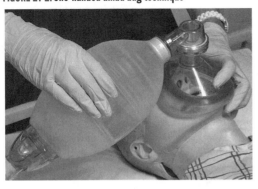

FIGURE 21-3: Two-handed ambu bag technique

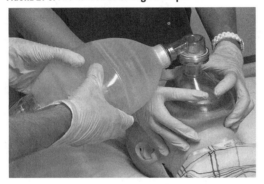

FIGURE 21-4: Macintosh blades

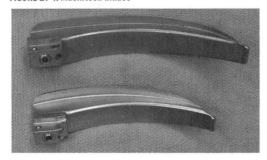

FIGURE 21-5: Miller blades

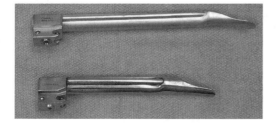

- If using a Miller blade, advance blade to the epiglottis and lift the epiglottis upward toward the ceiling to view vocal cords and glottis opening (examples of Miller blades are in **FIGURE 21-5**).
- Confirm visualization of vocal cords (glottis opening).
- With the right hand, insert ETT into the right corner of the mouth, through the vocal cords, and into the trachea.
- After ETT cuff passes the vocal cords, remove stylet (if used), and advance ETT to distance of approximately 22 cm at the lip.
- Inflate ETT cuff with a minimum amount of air to seal the trachea.
- Squeeze BVM to deliver positive pressure ventilation.
- Confirm ETT placement by auscultating bilateral breath sounds and negative gastric sounds over the abdomen and by confirming positive $ETCO_2$ (see **FIGURE 21-6**). Adjust ETT position as needed.
- Once proper position is confirmed, secure ETT in place with tape.

AFTERCARE INSTRUCTIONS

- If endotracheal intubation is not successful and the patient is rapidly deteriorating, a supraglottic airway device such as a laryngeal mask airway (LMA) may be used to temporarily ventilate the patient if BVM ventilation is not effective.
- If unable to intubate patient using conventional method as noted under procedural instructions, a **video laryngoscope** (e.g., GlideScope) may be utilized.[5,6]
  - Hold the GlideScope in the left hand and insert the blade midline into the patient's mouth.
  - Watching the video screen, advance blade until visualization of the glottic opening is obtained.
  - Insert ETT into the right side of the mouth and advance through the glottic opening, watching the video screen to guide proper placement (see **FIGURE 21-7**).

FIGURE 21-6: Endotracheal tube

Proper Endotracheal Intubation

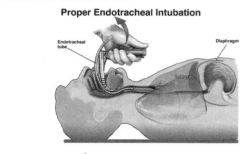

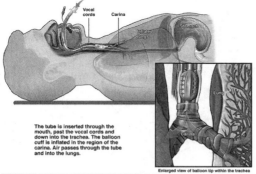

The tube is inserted through the mouth, past the vocal cords and down into the trachea. The balloon cuff is inflated in the region of the carina. Air passes through the tube and into the lungs.

Enlarged view of balloon tip within the trachea

© Nucleus Medical Art Inc / Alamy Stock Photo

FIGURE 21-7: Endotracheal tube placement

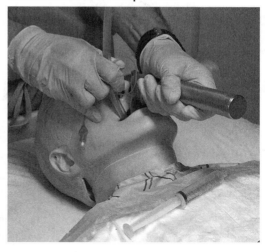

- Once ETT has been placed and proper placement verified (auscultating bilateral breath sounds, negative gastric sounds over the abdomen, and confirming positive $ETCO_2$), a chest x-ray is obtained to confirm correct anatomic location.

► REFERENCES

1. Wang HE, Kupas DF, Greenwood MJ, et al. An algorithmic approach to prehospital airway management. *Prehosp Emerg Care.* 2005;9(2):145–155.
2. Thomas E, Moss S. Tracheal intubation. *Anaesth Intens Care.* 2010;10(11):410–412.
3. Dorsch JA, Dorsch SE. Tracheal tubes and associated equipment. In: *Understanding Anesthesia Equipment.* 5th ed. Philadelphia, PA: Lippincott Williams & Wilkins; 2011: 561–632.
4. Stackhouse R, Infosino A. Airway management. In: Miller R, Pardo M, eds., *Basics of Anesthesia.* 6th ed. Philadelphia, PA: Elsevier Saunders; 2011: 219–251.
5. Heiner J, Gabot M. Airway management. In: Nagelhout J, Plaus K, eds., *Nurse Anesthesia.* 5th ed. Philadelphia, PA: Elsevier Saunders; 2014: 423–469.
6. Stewart CE. Tracheal intubation. In: *Advanced Airway Management.* Upper Saddle River NJ: Pearson Education; 2002: 76–113.
7. Morgan GE, Mikhail MM. Airway management. In: *Clinical Anesthesiology.* 5th ed. New York, NY: McGraw-Hill Lang; 309–341.
8. Grover A, Canavan C. Tracheal intubation. *Anaesth Intens Care.* 2007;8(9);347–351.
9. Rosenblatt W, Sukhupragarn W. Airway management. In Barash PG, Cullen BF, Stoetling RK, et al. eds. *Clinical Anesthesia.* 7th ed. Philadelphia, PA: Lippincott Williams & Wilkins; 2013;762–802.

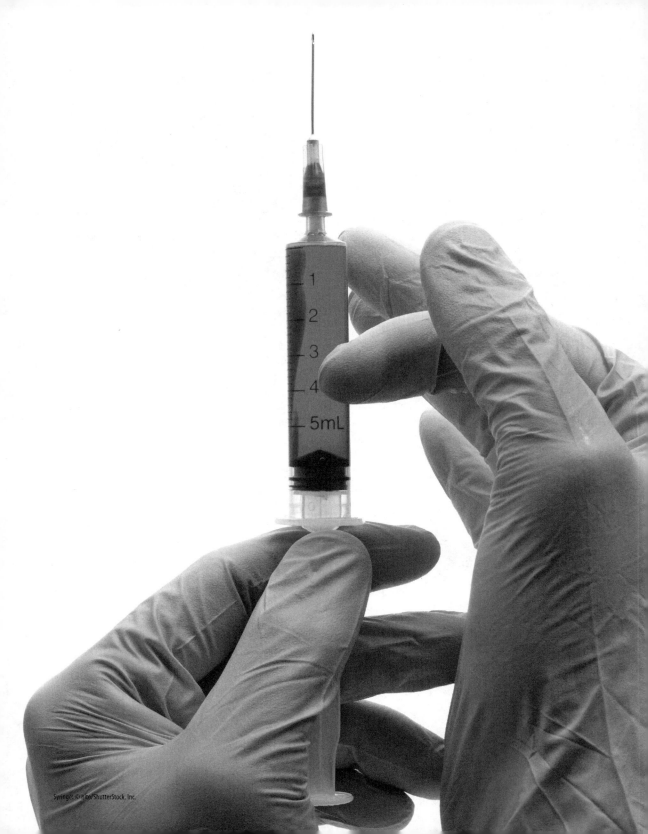

CHAPTER 22

Ventilator Management

Nikhil Chawla, MD
Michael Green, DO

GOAL

▶ Initiate, monitor, and adjust a mechanical ventilator according to the patient's response and medical condition.

OBJECTIVES

1. Understand the rationale for the need of mechanical ventilation and its necessity in certain situations.
2. Adequately identify indications for use of ventilators.
3. Acknowledge the multitude of ventilator settings and use them to appropriately manage the patient.
4. Delineate the various modes of conventional ventilators.
5. Initiate mechanical ventilation in patients by becoming well versed with setup and additional therapies required to effectively administer the therapy.
6. Identify the various complications that arise with the use of ventilators, including recognizing the early signs and treatment of any such iatrogenic injury.

RATIONALE FOR PROCEDURE

- Although the idea of mechanical ventilation has been around for nearly 400 years, it was around the polio epidemic of 1955 that widespread use of assisted ventilation gained traction. It was not long before prototype positive pressure lung inflation devices were being used at Massachusetts General Hospital and achieved widespread success. The ability to ventilate patients with respiratory distress and numerous other pathologies ushered in the era of critical care.
- The need for mechanical ventilation in critically ill patients cannot be emphasized enough, especially in cases where even temporary usage of assisted ventilation may help the patient over the proverbial "hump." While newer, noninvasive strategies of management of ventilation have come up, conventional ventilators have remained the gold standard for management of patients with respiratory distress.
- Mechanical ventilation is a lifesaving therapeutic modality but is only supposed to be a temporary solution. It is completely opposite from normal ventilatory physiology and therefore poses some unique risks to the patient. The best mode of ventilation is the one that has the fewest adverse effects. In brief, treating the underlying cause of illness should be the priority.

EVIDENCE-BASED INDICATIONS

- Although there are numerous reasons for the use of assisted ventilation, the following are the more common:
  - Respiratory failure
  - Cardiopulmonary arrest
  - Trauma, especially involving head, neck, and chest
  - Cardiovascular collapse
  - Shock (neurologic, septic, and cardiogenic)
  - Neurologic impairment (seizures, drugs, stroke)
  - Pulmonary pathologies (infections, tumors, bleeding, pneumothorax)
- These indications are by no means all inclusive and decisions regarding initiating ventilation should be made on a case-by-case basis. The decision to place a patient on mechanical ventilation is always a difficult one to make, but remember that an elective intubation, compared to emergency, carries with it less chances of something going wrong. Thus, if a patient's condition is severe enough to consider ventilation, proceed without delay.

BASICS OF VENTILATORS

Before dealing with complexities of the various modes of ventilation, it is important to be well versed with the various settings seen on the modern-day ventilators. The following are a few settings:

- Fraction of inspired oxygen (FiO_2): Defined as the percentage of oxygen in the inhaled gas. It can be adjusted up and down to provide adequate oxygenation to the patient.
- Respiratory rate: Usually set as breaths/minute.
- **Tidal volume**: Volume to be given with every breath.
- I:E ratio: The ratio of inspiratory and expiratory times during the respiratory cycle. The most commonly used ratio is 1:2.
- Peak pressure limit: The minimum pressure at which the ventilator will terminate the breath to avoid barotrauma to the lungs.
- Positive end-expiratory pressure (PEEP): Defined as the airway pressure at the end of expiration. It works to prevent the distal airways from collapsing on expiration. It is also helpful in recruitment of alveoli in patients with acute respiratory distress syndrome (ARDS) or acute lung injury.
- **Minute ventilation**: Calculated based on the tidal volumes and respiratory rate of the patient.

MODES OF VENTILATION

Since the 1960s, about 20 different modes of ventilation have been discovered. It is very daunting for new students to understand the technical details and uses of all these modes. The following are the most commonly used modes:

1. *Assist-control ventilation (ACV)*: This is the most commonly used mode of ventilation. It involves the use of a constant inflation volume instead of constant pressure. This mode allows the patient to initiate each mechanical breath (assisted ventilation) but will deliver a preset number of breaths if the patient's respiratory rate falls below the set limit (controlled ventilation). This mode has often been postulated to have the most effect on the **work of breathing** by assisting with every breath the patient initiates, but evidence indicates there is little impact on the work of breathing.[1] The *disadvantages* of using this mode are:
   - **Volutrauma** associated with use of higher than normal tidal volumes (12–15 mL/kg), a practice that has lost its footing in recent years. Recent studies have shown improved outcomes in patients with lung injury, with low volume (6 mL/kg) lung-protective ventilation.[2]
   - Auto-PEEP is a problem encountered in patients who are breathing at a rapid rate, which does not allow for the adequate time for exhaling; this leads to air entrapment and causes increased airway pressures after expiration.

2. *Intermittent mandatory ventilation (IMV)*: This mode was developed to overcome the shortcomings of ACV in patients with rapid respiratory rates (especially neonates). It is designed to provide only partial support, with periods of ACV and periods during which the patient breathes spontaneously to prevent hyperinflation. The most commonly used variation of IMV is synchronized IMV, or SIMV. It involves synchronization of the assisted breaths with the patient's spontaneous breaths. The patient usually receives a set rate of assist breaths, and the rate is changed as needed. It is also a common practice now to use pressure-support ventilation (described later in this chapter) during the spontaneous breathing periods. This has been shown to decrease the work of breathing[3] and improve patient tolerance. The *disadvantages* of using IMV are:
   - Increased work of breathing due to spontaneous breathing through a high-resistance circuit. The addition of pressure support has minimized this as discussed previously.
   - Decreased cardiac output in patients with left ventricular dysfunction by increasing the afterload.[4]

3. *Pressure-controlled ventilation (PCV)*: This mode uses a predetermined constant pressure to inflate the lung instead of constant volume, as is used in ACV and IMV. Although PCV can lead to variable tidal volumes, it might offer protection against ventilator-induced lung injury and decrease work of breathing. However, there is no evidence to support this claim.[5] The major disadvantage of PCV is variability of tidal volumes with changes in compliance of the lungs; therefore, it is better to use in patients with neurologic disorders with normal pulmonary compliance. A well-known modification of PCV is inverse ratio ventilation. This mode simply involves using a prolonged inspiration time compared to expiration—namely, an I:E ratio of 2:1 instead of the usual 1:2. Prolonged inspiration time allows for prevention of alveolar collapse, but at the same time increases the chances of developing auto-PEEP. The major indication of this mode is ARDS patients who have refractory hypoxemia.[6]

4. *Pressure support ventilation (PSV)*: This mode allows the patient to be able to determine the tidal volumes and respiratory time. PSV is a purely supportive mode of ventilation that provides a continuous pressure during the entire inspiration duration with

decelerating flows. Each breath is triggered when a negative pressure is generated by the patient and is terminated when the flow falls below 25% of the peak flow. Being a more physiologically acceptable method of positive pressure ventilation, PSV is used to decrease work of breathing when breathing spontaneously with high-resistance circuits. The common indications for its use are weaning off the ventilator and in conjunction with SIMV to reduce the work of breathing.

5. *Volume support ventilation (VSV)*: Just like PSV, this is also a supportive mode of ventilation. The ventilator delivers a preset tidal volume at a constant pressure with decelerating flows but the pressure varies from breath to breath. The major drawbacks of this mode are reduction of respiratory drive if the volume is set high and complicated settings that make them difficult to understand.

6. *Continuous positive airway pressure (CPAP)*: Maintenance of constant positive pressure throughout the respiratory cycle in a spontaneously breathing patient is known as CPAP. The patient does not need to generate a negative airway pressure to receive inhaled gas. It is a very commonly used technique for weaning off the ventilator as it decreases the work of breathing for a spontaneously breathing patient. It also has been established as the mode of choice for noninvasive positive pressure ventilation. CPAP has been used to successfully postpone intubation in patients with acute respiratory distress.[7] CPAP (especially nasal CPAP) is successfully being used in patients with known obstructive sleep apnea to keep the airway open during times of decreased upper airway muscle tone.

MONITORING OF VENTILATED PATIENT

- Patients requiring mechanical ventilation are usually critically ill and require meticulous continuous hemodynamic monitoring. Pulse oximetry, electrocardiogram (5 lead), noninvasive blood pressure, routine blood gas measurements, and ventilatory alarms are a minimum. A patient's condition might warrant more invasive monitoring in addition to the monitors previously mentioned. Of all these monitoring techniques, blood gas measurements are the single most important tool used to modify ventilator plans for patients. Hypoxia and hypercarbia, along with the serum pH, help titrate therapy. A patient with ongoing hypoxia can be managed by changing the FiO_2 or alveolar recruitment techniques, such as adding PEEP. Hypercarbia is best treated by increasing minute ventilation. Understanding of the utility of serum pH is more complex and depends on the type of abnormality the patient has. The ventilator is a very good tool to treat respiratory acidosis and can also be used in a compensatory way for metabolic acidosis. In cases of acid–base imbalance, it is imperative to treat the underlying pathology, because mechanical ventilation is at best a temporary measure.

- Most modern ventilators will allow for assessment of the patient's lung mechanics. Airway pressure measurements (end-expiratory peak and plateau pressures), thoracic compliance, and airway resistance are the commonly measured variables. These can be used not only to troubleshoot any ventilator alarms, but more importantly they act as diagnostic tools. Increased peak pressure signifies airway obstruction in the face of unchanged plateau pressure, but decreased compliance of the lung if plateau pressure is increased. Thoracic compliance is a good tool to monitor the progression of certain disease pathologies such as ARDS, wherein increasing compliance signifies improvement.

VENTILATOR EQUIPMENT

See **FIGURE 22-1**.

FIGURE 22-1: Oxygen ventilator

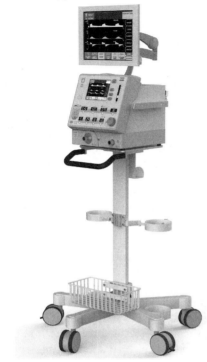

ADDITIONAL THERAPIES FOR VENTILATED PATIENTS

- Positive pressure delivery requires establishment of airway with plastic endotracheal tubes or tracheostomy tubes. These tubes usually have a cuff that is inflated to seal the trachea and prevent leakage of pressure to the environment. Using these airway devices necessitates regular checks to avoid malfunction. Routine chest x-rays should be performed to confirm the positioning. The ideal position is the tip located 3–5 cm above the carina with the head in the neutral position. Due to their length, these airway devices provide increased resistance to airflow, and thus increase the work of breathing in a spontaneously ventilating patient. In general, the endotracheal tube diameter should be at least 7 mm in adults (preferably 8 mm) to reduce the influence on the airway resistance. Cuff leaks are common and should be treated to maintain the seal. The pressure in the cuff should not exceed 25 mmHg to avoid ischemic injury to the tracheal epithelium.[8] Recent use of high-volume, low-pressure cuffs has decreased the risk of pressure-induced injury.

- Routine suctioning should be a standard practice in patients who are intubated. Intubation and ventilation decrease patients' ability to clear secretions and puts them at higher risk for aspiration. Contrary to popular belief, recent evidence shows cuff inflation does not protect against aspiration. Elevation of the head above the bed and regular suctioning are good practices to prevent aspiration. Other therapies such as gastric tubes and gastric acid prophylaxis have not been shown to be helpful; gastric tubes might actually increase the risk of aspiration. Additionally, oral care and brushing of teeth help to prevent ventilator-associated pneumonia (VAP).

- Ventilation usually necessitates use of pharmacological adjuvants to be efficacious. Intubated patients will usually require sedation to reduce discomfort, alleviate anxiety, facilitate ventilation, and improve oxygenation, unless precluded by the medical condition. The most commonly used medications are benzodiazepines, propofol, and dexmedetomidine. Whenever sedating a ventilated patient, consideration must be given to the use of opioids to provide analgesia. Neuromuscular blocking agents might be considered in certain circumstances to decrease the work of breathing and to improve oxygenation, although the data regarding use of paralytics remain conflicting.

COMPLICATIONS

- Although mechanical ventilation is a lifesaving modality, it comes with its own associated risks.

- A patient undergoing positive pressure ventilation is at an increased risk of aspiration. Aspiration precaution strategies such as patient positioning and regular suctioning have been discussed earlier in the chapter. The increased aspiration risk and inability to clear tracheal secretions can lead to VAP, a dreaded complication that needs to be tackled early and vigorously with broad-spectrum antibiotics, respiratory toilet, and chest physical therapy.

- Some of the complications can be attributed to the mechanical effects of intubation and positive pressure on the lungs and airways.

- Increased cuff pressures and long-term intubation can cause tracheal mucosal ischemia, leading to tracheal stenosis later in life. Using too much volume in the cuff might dislodge the tube and cause damage to the vocal cords as well as hoarseness of voice.

- High tidal volumes and high peak pressures can cause barotrauma and lead to acute lung injury. Clinically apparent alveolar rupture is the ultimate expression in the spectrum of acute lung injury. It can present as subcutaneous or mediastinal emphysema. If the rupture involves the visceral pleura, a pneumothorax may result.

- The effects of positive pressure on cardiac output are complex. It usually will lead to decreased preload and impede venous return by abolishing intrathoracic negative pressure developed while breathing spontaneously. Ventricular septal shift and decreased cardiac compliance due to positive pressure on the ventricular wall also compound this effect. At the same time, afterload is decreased as the positive pressure helps with the emptying of the ventricle. Addition of PEEP worsens the preload and can cause a decrease in cardiac output, especially in patients who are hypovolemic to begin with.

- Immobility associated with intubation and sedation puts patients at risk for deep venous thrombosis, pressure ulcers, and fluid retention. Stress ulcers are seen frequently.

- Long-term intubation and sedation might put the patient at risk for inadequate nutrition. Nutritional supplementation via the enteral or parenteral route should be established.

► REFERENCES

1. Marini JJ, Capps JS, Culver BH. The inspiratory work of breathing during assisted mechanical ventilation. *Chest.* 1985;87:612–618.
2. The Acute Respiratory Distress Syndrome Network. Ventilation with lower tidal volumes as compared with traditional volumes for acute lung injury and the acute respiratory distress syndrome. *N Engl J Med.* 2000;342:1301–1308.
3. Leung P, Jubran A, Tobin MJ. Comparison of assisted ventilator modes on triggering, patient effort, and dyspnea. *Am J Respir Crit Care Med.* 1997;155:194–1948.
4. Mathru M, Rao TL, El-Etr AA, et al. Hemodynamic responses to changes in ventilatory patterns in patients with normal and poor left ventricular reserve. *Crit Care Med.* 1982;10:423–426.
5. Kallet RH, Campbell AR, Dicker RA, et al. Work of breathing during lung-protective ventilation in patients with acute lung injury and acute respiratory distress syndrome: a comparison between volume and pressure-regulated breathing modes. *Respir Care.* 2005;50(12):1623–1631.
6. Wang SH, Wei TS. The outcome of early pressure-controlled inverse ratio ventilation on patients with severe acute respiratory distress syndrome in surgical intensive care unit. *Am J Surg.* 2001;183:151–155.
7. Brochard L, Mancebo J, Elliott MW. Noninvasive ventilation for acute respiratory failure. *Eur Respir J.* 2002;19:712–721.
8. Heffner JE, Hess D. Tracheostomy management in the chronically ventilated patient. *Clin Chest Med.* 2001;22:561–568.

GLOSSARY

actinic keratosis   Potentially precancerous lesion that can turn into squamous cell skin cancer. Rough, scaly white to pink macules or papules.

aerobic bacteria   Bacteria that require oxygen in order to survive (e.g., *Staphylococcus* species, *Streptococcus* species, *Enterobacteriaceae* species, and *Mycobacterium tuberculosis*).

air embolism   Bubbles of air in the cardiac or vascular system that result from trauma and create an obstruction.

airway assessment   Evaluation of a person's mouth opening, quality of dentition, tongue size, neck circumference, and cervical mobility to determine the degree of ease to perform an intubation.

Allen test   A test in which the patient is asked to clench his or her hand into a fist. Afterward, the provider puts pressure on both the radial and ulnar arteries, then releases to observe blood flow to determine if either artery is occluded.

amide   A compound with an organic functional group containing a carbonyl group linked to a nitrogen atom.

anaerobic bacteria   Bacteria that can thrive in an environment in which there is little or no oxygen (e.g., *Clostridium tetani*, *Escherichia coli*, and *Klebsiella* species).

analgesia   Absence of sensation to painful stimuli.

anesthesia   Absence of sensation or feeling.

aponeurosis   Layers of flat, broad tendons.

arterial puncture   A medical procedure in which a needle is inserted into the radial artery with no exposure to air in order to determine radial blood gas values.

asepsis   The absence of pathogens—bacteria, viruses, or other microorganisms—to protect against infection.

aseptic technique   The practice of incorporating sterile precautionary measures to prevent contamination of a person, object, or area during a procedure.

aspiration   The act of pulling back the plunger of the syringe once the needle has been inserted to observe for blood as an indication of improper injection placement.

bacteremia   The presence of bacteria in the blood.

basic airway management   Performance of a simple maneuver such as a chin lift/jaw thrust or insertion of an oral/nasal airway to alleviate upper airway obstruction.

bladder   A distensible, hollow, and muscular organ that collects urine from the kidneys.

Carson catheter   A Coudé-tipped catheter designed to navigate the neck of the bladder in female patients and the urethra of male patients with a stricture or benign prostatic hypertrophy.

catheter   A flexible, tubular instrument that is inserted into a body cavity in order to remove fluid; most often inserted into the bladder to drain urine.

central nervous system   Bodily system representing the brain and spinal cord.

cerebrospinal fluid   Clear fluid produced in choroid plexus of the cerebral ventricles, surrounds the spinal cord and brain.

chevron taping   A method to tape a catheter in place with a crisscross V-shaped pattern to stabilize it.

chlorhexidine   An antiseptic agent used to clean a patient's skin prior to an injection or other procedure.

choanal atresia   Blockage of back of nasal passage.

chylothorax   Lymphatic fluid in the pleural cavity.

closed fracture   Also known as a simple fracture; the bone does not break the skin.

coagulopathic   Failure of clotting system to form clots in order to prevent bleeding.

compartment syndrome   Increased pressure in the fascial layers of muscle.

Coudé-tipped catheter   A catheter with a slightly curved (bent), rigid tip that is used to navigate past obstructions in the urinary tract; examples are enlarged prostates in men or urethral scarring in women.

Council-tip stylet   A metal guidewire that provides stiffness to a catheter and has a screw tip on the end that is most often used to treat acute retention in emergency situations.

diabetic ketoacidosis (DKA)   A life-threatening condition in patients with diabetes in which the body uses fat for fuel due to lack of insulin and as a result produces too many ketones (waste by-product of fat).

dialysis shunt   A connection between a vein and an artery; fistula.

diffusing capacity of the lungs for carbon monoxide (DLCO)   Measures the ability of the lungs to transfer gas from inhaled air to the red blood cells in the pulmonary capillaries.

ectocervix   The visible area of the cervix that is covered with squamous epithelium.

electrocardiogram (ECG or EKG)   A printed representation of the electrical activity of the heart by recording the primary electrical event of contraction and the recovery phase of the myocardial tissue limb leads.

empyema   Collection of inflammatory fluid and miscellaneous substances.

endocervix   The opening of the cervix that leads to the uterus.

endotracheal intubation   The insertion of an artificial airway into the trachea to deliver positive pressure ventilation and protect the lungs against aspiration.

epiglottis   An elastic cartilage flap attached to the base of the tongue, which covers the glottis during swallowing to prevent aspiration of food or liquid.

esophageal stricture   Narrowing of the esophagus.

ester   A compound containing a carboxylic acid linked to an O-alkyl group.

extravasation   Accidental leakage of IV fluid into the extravascular space or tissues surrounding the IV insertion site.

fascia   Connective tissue fibers—primarily collagen—that form bands under the skin to attach, separate, and stabilize muscles and other organ structures.

fenestrated drape   A drape sheet used in medical procedures that has a slit-like opening or window to expose an anatomic area.

FiO$_2$ Fraction of inspired oxygen concentration.

Fitzpatrick skin typing   A system to categorize skin color, pigmentation, risk of sunburn, and risk of scarring developed by Thomas Fitzpatrick, MD.

Foley catheter   A sterile and flexible tube passed through the urethra to drain the bladder. It is the most common type of indwelling catheter.

forced expiratory volume (FEV1)   Total volume of air that a patient can exhale in 1 second after a full inspiration; it is affected by airway resistance. The FEV1 falls approximately 30 mL (cc) per year.

forced vital capacity (FVC)   Total volume of air that a patient can exhale after a full inspiration; it is reduced in diseases that cause the lungs to be smaller. Overall accuracy of the FVC for restriction is about 60%.

French   Abbrevated as Fr; the measurement system used to refer to the size of a catheter's circumference. A unit is 3 times the diameter in millimeters—equivalent to 0.33 millimeters or 0.013 inches.

healthcare-associated infections   Infections acquired during a hospital stay or during an outpatient procedure, regardless of the mechanism or cause.

hematoma   Bruise causing a collection of blood.

hemochromatosis   An accumulation of iron in the blood from any cause.

hemopneumothorax   Blood and air in the pleural cavity.

hemothorax   Blood in the pleural cavity.

heparinized blood gas syringe   A syringe that has been prepared with heparin to act as an anticoagulant, used for drawing blood gas samples.

hydrothorax   Serous fluid accumulation in the pleural cavity.

indwelling catheter   A catheter that is left inside the body for a period of time—either temporarily or permanently; it is often used for urinary incontinence.

infiltration   The accumulation of fluid that is not normal or in excess of normal amount

inflammatory phase   The body's natural response to an injury, which lasts from day 1 of the injury to day 5 post-injury. It involves pain, erythema, and edema.

inotrope   A medication that modifies the force or speed of muscle contraction.

ischemia   Restriction in blood supply to tissues causing a shortage of oxygen and glucose to tissues needed to keep cells viable.

joint dislocation   Abnormal separation of the bones in a joint.

keloid   An overgrowth of fibrous tissue that extends beyond the margins of a wound.

laryngospasm   Sudden and forceful closure of the vocal cords blocking the flow of oxygen into the lungs.

lipohypertrophy   Buildup of subcutaneous tissue at a continuously used insulin injection site.

lumbar puncture   Also called spinal tap, insertion of spinal needle between two vertebrae into subarachnoid space to remove CSF for pressure decrease or diagnosis of infection and other disorders.

lymphedema   A non-pitting form of lymph fluid buildup in tissue due to an a lymphatic obstruction.

metabolic acidosis   A pH imbalance in which the body produces excessive acid or the kidneys are unable to remove acid at an adequate rate.

metabolic alkalosis   A pH imbalance in which there is an increase in serum bicarbonate concentration and the pH of the body's tissue rises above the normal range.

methemoglobinemia   A disorder characterized by an elevated presence of ferric rather than ferrous hemoglobin in the blood.

minute ventilation   Total breaths volume over a 1-minute interval.

monitor electrodes   Small disks that are attached to a patient's chest, connected to precordial leads, during an ECG.

myelin   Material forming a layer of insulation around a neuronal axon, which speeds up transmission of impulses.

myocardial hypertrophy   A disease of the heart muscle in which the muscle is oxygen-deprived and becomes thick with impaired function.

myocardial infarction   A sudden and sometimes fatal occurrence of coronary thrombosis, typically resulting in the death of part of a heart muscle.

myocardial ischemia   Restriction of blood flow and oxygen to the heart muscle; often caused by an arterial blockage.

negative depolarization   Any electrical activity that moves away from the positive electrode.

non-retention catheter   A type of straight catheter with lumen at tip and end that is designed for short-term urine drainage.

Occupational Safety and Health Administration   An office of the U.S. government tasked with ensuring the health and safety of men and women at their places of work.

onychomycosis   Fungal infection of the nail.

open fracture   The affected bone(s) break the skin.

peaked expiratory flow rate (PEFR)   A measurement of how fast a patient can exhale; often used in asthma patients.

personal protective equipment (PPE)   Equipment worn by healthcare professionals, designed to protect the person from exposure to workplace pathogens or biohazards.

phlebitis   Inflammation of the vein walls, often the superficial veins, commonly caused by one or more blood clots. Signs include warmth, tenderness, and erythema.

plaster of Paris   Gypsum plaster (anhydrous calcium sulfate) used in bandages to protect limbs and broken bones.

pneumothorax   A collection of air or gas in the pleural space that can cause part or all of a lung to collapse.

polycythemia vera   A neoplasia of the bone marrow resulting in overproduction of red blood cells.

positive depolarization   Any electrical activity that moves toward the positive electrode.

precordial leads   The 6 unipolar chest leads used in an ECG, in which positive electrodes are placed in a horizontal plane over the heart.

preoxygenation   The administration of 100% high-flow oxygen via facemask to replace the nitrogen in the lungs with oxygen.

proliferative phase   A wound healing phase characterized by fibroblast proliferation stimulated by macrophage-released growth factors; increased rate of collagen synthesis by fibroblasts, granulation tissue, and neovascularization; and gain in tensile strength. It lasts approximately 72 hours to 6 weeks post injury.

pseudocholinesterase   An enzyme present in the blood responsible for hydrolyzing acetylcholine.

pyogenic granuloma   Benign vascular neoplasm.

Quincke needle   A type of spinal needle with cutting tip.

radial artery   A branch of the brachial artery that supplies blood to the hand.

remodeling phase   This wound healing phase starts approximately 6 weeks after the wound occurs and may last 1 year post-injury. This phase is characterized by an increase in tensile strengths; scar flattens and loses its red appearance.

Robinson catheter   A type of non-retention catheter that is straight with lumen at tip and end used for short-term urine drainage.

seborrheic keratosis   Benign growths that develop due to age. These lesions can be flesh colored, uneven, multiple colors of brown, and with a variegated wart-like surface.

Seldinger technique   A special method of placing a catheter into a blood vessel by passing over a guidewire.

Silastic catheter   A catheter with a smooth silicone exterior that is designed as an indwelling catheter with a large drainage lumen that can be left in for extended periods of time; usually green.

silicone catheter   Similar to a Foley catheter, except it is more rigid; it is the only latex-free catheter, so is ideal for patients with a latex allergy.

skin antisepsis   Creating a pathogen-free environment on a person's skin in preparation for a medical procedure.

sniffing position   Head extension that aligns the oral, pharyngeal, and laryngeal axes to obtain the best view of the glottis opening.

soft-tissue injury   Damage of ligaments, tendons, or muscles.

sprain   Stretching or tearing of a ligament.

Sprotte needle   A type of spinal needle with a pencil-point tip and side hole.

straight catheter   A type of non-retention catheter that is straight with lumen at tip and end for drainage.

stylet   A thin wire inserted into a hollow needle to give it rigidity and ensure patency.

supraglottic airway device   An airway tube such as a laryngeal mask airway (LMA) connected to an inflatable cuff that seals the hypopharynx and facilitates oxygen flow into the lungs.

swathe   To wrap or bandage.

synthetic plaster   Newer casting materials such as fiberglass and latex-free compounds that can be substituted for plaster of Paris to protect limbs and broken bones.

tendinopathy   A torn or painful tendon usually resulting from injury.

tenosynovitis   Inflammation of the tendon sheath often from overuse of affected tendon.

therapeutic phlebotomy   The practice of having blood drawn for the treatment of a disease.

three-way catheter   A type of Foley catheter that has three ports: a tube for drainage, a tube for balloon inflation, and a tube to instill irrigation fluid.

thrombophlebitis   Inflammation of the wall of a vein with associated thrombosis, often occurring in the legs during pregnancy.

tidal volume   Volume of air expired with every breath.

Tiemann catheter   A Coudé-tipped catheter designed to navigate the male urethra, especially when there is a stricture present.

tourniquet   A constricting or compressive device used to stop or slow down circulation.

transformation zone   The area of the cervix where squamous epithelium and columnar epithelium meet; squamocolumnar junction.

ultrasonographic guidance   Sound waves that produce an image to help guide diagnostic information.

urinary catheterization   The process of inserting a catheter into the bladder to drain urine.

urinary retention   An inability to completely empty one's bladder; thus, some amount of urine is "retained" in the bladder. Also known as ischuria.

urine   Liquid by-product of the body secreted by kidneys.

vallecula   A space between the base of the tongue and the epiglottis where the Macintosh laryngoscope blade is inserted.

vascular device   Any device that has obtained access to the vasculature (e.g., intravenous cannulas typically placed in the extremities, peripherally inserted central catheter [PICC], central line in the subclavian vein or femoral vein, or a venous port inserted into the chest wall).

vasodilator   A drug that causes the dilation of blood vessels.

vasopressor   A drug that causes the constriction of blood vessels.

vasopressors   Medications used to constrict blood vessels.

venipuncture   Process of obtaining intravenous access for the purpose of intravenous therapy or for blood sampling of venous blood.

venous sample A sample of deoxygenated blood taken from a vein.

video laryngoscope A video or optically based laryngoscope, which projects the view onto a screen, allowing the clinician to visualize the glottic opening.

volutrauma Lung injury caused as a result of excessively high ventilator volumes.

Whitacre needle A type of spinal needle with a type pencil-point tip and side hole that is smaller than the side hole in a Sprotte needle.

work of breathing Effort required to inflate the lungs—usually 5% of total body energy expenditure but can increase significantly with critical illness.

Zenker diverticulum Esophageal pouch that develops in the upper esophagus.

Index

H

HAIs. *See* healthcare-associated infections
hand antisepsis, 11*t*
hand care, types of, 10, 11*t*
handwashing, 10–11, 10*f*, 11*f*, 11*t*, 18
healthcare-associated infections (HAIs), 4
    handwashing, 10–11, 10*f*, 11*f*, 11*t*
hearing impairment, 155
hemochromatosis, 62
hemorrhage, 154–155
hemostasis, 114
hemothorax, 128, 163
heparinized blood gas syringe, 48
high-grade squamous intraepithelial lesions (HSILs),
    123–124
horizontal mattress suture, suture placement for, 87*f*
hydrothorax, 128
hypercarbia, 178
hypoxia, 178

I

I:E ratio, 176
immunoglobulins, 157
IMV. *See* intermittent mandatory ventilation
inadvertent catheterization of vaginal canal, 30
indwelling catheters, 28, 34–35
    care of, 35
    removal of, 35–36
infiltration, 40
inflammatory phase of wound healing, 84
injections
    intradermal injections, 56–57
    intramuscular injections, 55–56
    subcutaneous injections, 57–58
inotropes, 160
insertion techniques, nasogastric tube placement, 22–25,
    22*f*–24*f*
intercostal neuralgia, 128–129
intermittent mandatory ventilation (IMV), 177
internal jugular vein, 143
intradermal injections, 56–57
intraepithelial lesion, 123
intramuscular injections, 55–56
invasive cancer, 124*f*
IV cannulation, 41

IV fluid, 42, 42*f*
IV insertion, 40–44, 41*f*–44*f*
    tourniquet and insert IV catheter, 42*f*
    vascular access supplies, 41*f*

J

jaw thrust, 170–171, 171*f*
jugular vein, 163

L

lactate, 157
laryngeal mask airway (LMA), 172–173
laryngospasm, 170
lead placement, 73*f*
lidocaine, 49*f*, 106, 151, 152*f*
lidocaine infiltration, 136
limb leads, 73
lipohypertrophy, 54
liquid-based Pap cytology test, 122
liquid nitrogen cryosurgery. *See* cryotherapy
LMA. *See* laryngeal mask airway
local anesthesia, 102–106, 104*f*
    anesthetic vial for, 151, 152*f*
longitudinal biopsy, 112, 113
low-grade squamous intraepithelial lesions (LSILs), 123
lower leg splint, 96*f*
lumbar puncture, 150–157, 151*f*, 152*f*, 157*t*
    pediatric, 155–156
lung capacities, 79
lung volumes, 79, 79*f*
lunula, 112

M

males
    anchor drainage bag, 34, 35*f*
    cleanse urethral meatus, 33
    insert catheter, 33–34
    urinary catheter insertion, 32, 33
malignancy, 123
manometer, 151, 151*f*
masks, 9, 9*f*
mechanical ventilation, 176
medical emergency oxygen station, 179*f*
melanomas, 112
methemoglobinemia, 103

Index continued

Index continued